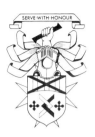

The Slipped Disc and the Aching Back of Man

by

ALEXANDER WALKER-NADDELL
FRCS, FRCPS, FSA Scot., FRSA, K.St.J, ERD, JP, DL
Consultant Orthopaedic and Neuro Surgeon

Edited by —
ANNIE E. LIVESEY MA

Illustrated by —
JUNE TAYLOR BA and KEN TAYLOR Des.RCA

Published by —
J. R. REID PRINTERS LTD., BLANTYRE, GLASGOW

Typeset in 10 point English Times
on Compugraphic MCS8400 Phototypesetter

ISBN 0 948785 00 4

Typeset, Printed and Published in Scotland by
J. R. Reid Printers Ltd., Blantyre, Glasgow.

Foreword

By STANLEY BAXTER

I ARRIVED in Glasgow still trailing my right leg. Sciatica stemming from back trouble had begun on a coast to coast tour of America. An American chiropractor, a distinguished Harley Street consultant and two osteopaths all had had a go at putting it right. Now I was two weeks away from opening night and hardly able to walk, never mind dance and clown around with Ronnie Corbett, as my role in 'Cinderella' demanded. When moaning about it to Herbert Lumsden, the theatre manager (I don't suffer in silence), Herbert said 'Oh, you ought to go to a fellow we've got in Glasgow. Max Bygraves had back trouble and this fellow put him right in no time.'

'Oh Herbert' I said 'I've done EVERYTHING. It's no use.'
'Well at least give him a try.'
'What's his name?'
'Walker-Naddell.'
'Sounds like pure quack. Double barrelled name . . .' my voice trailed off as another knife seared down the nerve in the right leg. Oh! God!! Alright! One more try. Where does he practise?'
'Sandyford Place.'

After a short wait I was ushered into a cosy old-fashioned consulting room, where I was greeted in a gruff, though friendly, voice by a sturdy muscular man of medium height. I told him the medical history and was astonished — almost angered — to hear him say, avuncularly, and with a confidence I regarded as verging on the insane, 'Oh we'll have you dancing by the end of the week!' I growled a trifle ruefully, 'Will you indeed?' and ticked off the list of miracle workers at whose hand I had suffered to no avail. Warming to my theme I added, 'One of your Harley Street colleagues even had me on a rack being stretched by two Amazons. I rounded off my tirade by saying 'Frankly I'm a mite cynical about these and even your orthopaedic colleagues'. *'You're* cynical? We'll shake on that sentiment' he rejoined, proferring a hand with the largest thumb protruding from it that I had ever seen. 'I'm a fully qualified orthopaedic surgeon myself but I seldom operate nowadays for this condition. It's done with the hands — and the exercises that I'll give you.'

A very brief session followed during which the famous thumb found the offending disc and detached it. I was manipulated briefly and given one simple exercise to do twice a day. There were two more visits before Walker-Naddell took me off his books but, as I stepped out into Sandyford Place that day, I knew already I'd found my saviour. And he was right about the dancing. I was 'charlestoning' with nary a twinge before the end of rehearsals.

Any time since that memorable occasion that I've twisted an ankle or sprained a back I've rushed back to 'WN' and he's never let me down. The last time I visited him he was telling me that an Arab Sheik had developed back trouble in London and a source not a thousand miles from the Foreign Office had got in touch with him, urging him to hasten south to treat the Middle Eastern V.I.P. 'So you had to go to London?' I said. 'Not I! I told them to send him up to Glasgow and get him in to a local hotel.'

In the pause that followed I looked out at a darkening Sauchiehall Street with thoughtful bemusement. He broke the silence with, 'You mustn't indulge these multi-millionaires y' know!'

Acknowledgements

IT HAS been my intention for many years to describe my technique for the treatment of a slipped disc and record the results of my treatment. At last, despite the daily commitments of a busy life that have delayed it and perhaps a little of that human frailty, procrastination, this intention has been fulfilled.

Its realisation has been achieved with the help of various people to whom I should like to express my sincere thanks. During my early years of research into this condition the late Mr. George H. Stevenson ("Stevie") former Senior General and Orthopaedic Surgeon to the Glasgow Royal Infirmary, was unfailing in his inspiration and encouragement of my work and I remember him not only with gratitude, but also with warmth and affection.

This book, based on 10 years of research in Glasgow Pathology Department, is the result of 30 years of experience and continuous assessment and improvement of my technique. Within recent times, Nan Livesey has worked with me on the book, helped me to structure it and express my ideas clearly and simply. It is difficult to describe a medical condition professionally with academic precision and at the same time make it intelligible to all readers from whatever walk of life they may come. I hope we have, in part, succeeded in doing this.

In order to present the whole picture as clearly as possible it was my idea to illustrate each aspect of the subject with an appropriate diagram on the opposite page of the text for easy reference. My thanks are due to Ken Taylor who with painstaking care transformed my own sketches into illustrations of a particularly high standard.

Finally, John R. Reid, despite all the vicissitudes that seem to be associated with publishing in this economic climate, overcame all obstacles in his path and finally put my words into print. His highly professional standard of printing from the outset saved many hours of correction.

To my grandchildren:
Dean, Beverley, Emma, Ian, Iris,
James and Anne

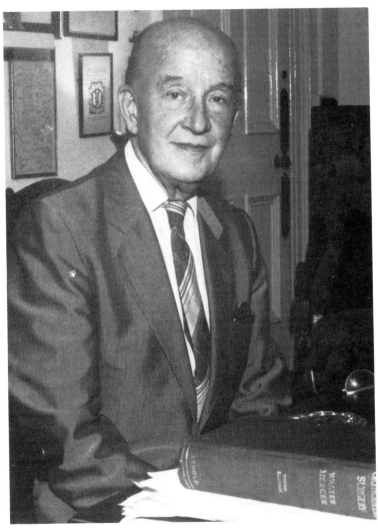

The Author

CONTENTS

Introduction

THE CONDITION of the slipped disc has always been present in man but the awareness of it has existed only during the last five decades. It is such a common and crippling condition that the term 'slipped disc' has become a household term. This widespread usage has, however, resulted in much confusion often revealing a basic misunderstanding about the condition and often stemming from a lack of accurate knowledge about the anatomy of the spinal column. For example, most patients visualise a disc as a piece of bone or cartilage which can slip in or out from its position between two opposing vertebral bodies and that the doctor or consultant will put the disc back into place to effect a cure. In actual fact, the disc is not bone or cartilage but made up of a jelly-like or myxomatous substance that cannot, because of its gelatinous nature, be pushed back into position, for it would simply disintegrate under pressure.

In order to provide a clear picture of the disc and its function and also to provide a sound basis for the promotion of my views about this condition, I have devoted the first two chapters of this book to a description of the spinal column and its nervous system. I have tried to present these anatomical details in simple terms for the benefit of lay readers. In addition, relevant new information, discovered during my years of research, is included and may be of interest to my medical colleagues.

A slipped disc condition occurs when the annular ligament that lies between any two opposing vertebral bodies and that surrounds the disc, becomes so weak either through injury or a summation of minor injuries, that a tear develops in it. This tear in the annular ligament allows the disc to prolapse and, if this protruding disc strikes a nerve root, the painful symptoms of a slipped disc condition are experienced.

We know that this condition is not a 'killer' disease, but it can destroy the quality of life, for the individual who suffers from it may be in constant agony, or in constant fear of agony. It can lead to severe incapacity and the number of man hours lost from work on account of this problem is very great. It occurs in people from all walks of life, for it is no respecter of persons. It can strike the chairman of a factory, just as severely as a member of his work force. In fact, the man who uses his back muscles, keeping them strong and in good tone, is actually less likely to develop a slipped disc lesion, unless, of course, he undergoes a severe accident to the spinal column.

Patients suffer terrible frustration of movement, may even become bedridden and yet, in many cases, doctors or even consultants, can find very little abnormality, for even straight x-rays often show negative results. In such circumstances, when a positive diagnosis is not made the patient becomes even more frustrated and sometimes, in extreme despair, he may turn for help outside the medical profession. In this book I have tried to build up diagnostic guidelines for complete and positive diagnosis of a disc lesion in every part of the spinal column and usually this diagnosis can be made without the use of x-ray.

However, when the symptoms do indicate a disc lesion condition, such a diagnosis often strikes fear into the heart of most patients, even in these days of advanced medical knowledge and techniques. Current text books provide little information about the condition itself, though they do give detailed methods of treatment including surgery, traction, surgical supports, the use of orthopaedic beds etc. Most of these methods, still widely used today, do not claim to effect a permanent cure but rather attempt to alleviate the symptoms. Only surgery claims to eliminate the disc itself, but most patients are quite naturally loathe to undergo this form of treatment, as the possible risks associated with it are great and often the final results are far from satisfactory. In Chapter VIII, I have tried to point out the merits and shortcomings of many of these methods of treatment.

Many, if not all, of these current methods still leave the patient unable to cope with heavy work and this could result in job loss or a change of employment. Most people, even after undergoing these treatments, have to adapt their lifestyle to cope with the weakness or residual discomfort in the back and are usually unable, any longer, to take part in any vigorous sport.

The vast number of differing methods must perhaps suggest there is no one satisfactory cure, and a great number of patients are known

10

to turn away, in pain and frustration, from the present prescribed methods of medical help. It is surely an indictment of the medical profession that such a state of affairs exists: that many people in despair, seek help from an unqualified practitioner. In one sense it is good in that the mystique that surrounds medicine should not be so strong that a layman should not question it, but, on the other hand, it behoves the medical profession to recognise the need for medically stable methods of treatment in this particular field, where many orthodox or current methods seem far from satisfactory.

Medicine is not an exact science but we, medical men, are constantly striving to make it so. However, there are many medical and surgical problems for which we do not have the complete answer. For a time, doctors will accept the current forms of treatment without question, even if the results are not completely effective. But man is a restless animal: a driving force within him leads him on to search for better ways of dealing with a specific problem. To this end, research plays a vital role and, at times, after a vast amount of experimental work in the laboratory, a new treatment is discovered. This may appear completely revolutionary, and therefore unacceptable to one's colleagues until it has been thoroughly proven.

In my treatment of the slipped disc I have evolved a completely new method, having copied no one in this field before me. I encountered opposition to it in my early years from my superiors and other medical colleagues. Nevertheless, as a qualified neuro- and orthopaedic surgeon, I have developed a method of diagnosis and treatment of the slipped disc which is the result of years of research in the Pathology Department of the Royal Infirmary of Glasgow, and the successful outcome of this treatment of literally thousands of patients has convinced me of the value of my method.

It became my sole aim to find a simple and effective way of curing a slipped disc lesion, and long research into the anatomy of the spinal column eventually convinced me of the true cause of the pain and resulted in a new, simple method of treatment. The fundamental part of the treatment is, quite briefly, the detaching of the spinal disc that is protruding through a tear in the annular ligament and mechanically pressing on a nerve root. This detachment is performed manually under a local anaesthetic. I call it the 'Non-Surgical Detachment of the Slipped Disc' and it is described in Chapters IV, V, VI and VII. Further treatment given includes 'surgical' manipulation to correct any deformity of the spinal column, that has arisen as a result of the disc lesion, and a specific Training Programme of exercises to regain tone in the affected muscle groups. I have attempted to describe it in terms any reader can understand, but also to include sufficient anatomical details to explain to my medical colleagues its viability and to give an exact description of my method of working.

Although a clear understanding of the anatomy of the spinal column and the function of the disc is beneficial to both patient and doctor, there may be readers whose prime concern is to learn simply about their own condition. They may, in this case, prefer to turn to Appendix II where the conditions of slipped disc lesions in the lumbar or lower back area, in the dorsal or chest area, in the cervical or neck area are separately described in summary form. Appendix II also contains an account of the treatment administered in the surgery and the set of exercises prescribed to further the cure. Advice is also given there on how to alleviate, and prevent any aggravation of, the symptoms during the period of recovery.

This book presents an entirely new form of treatment that in more than 90% of the cases treated over 30 years in my surgery in Glasgow has eradicated the condition of the slipped disc, allowing the patient to lead a normal life and also to take part in any form of sport, even at competitive level.

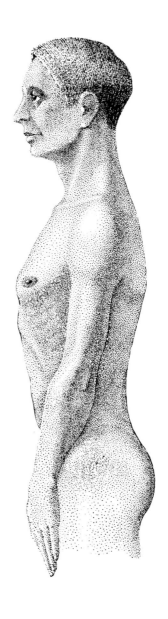

Diag. 1. Lateral view of the normal back.

14

CHAPTER I

The Development and Description of the Spinal Column

THOUGH MUCH of this chapter is familiar to all doctors, it is important, primarily for the benefit of readers not medically trained, to give a description of the development and structure of the various parts of the spinal column.

During the examination of a patient, the doctor or consultant always works from his knowledge of the healthy body, in order to recognise any malfunction or deformity in any part of the system. Thus a doctor must know the normal alignment of the spinal column and its relationship to the various muscle groups that control its movement. He must be able to recognise the normal contour of the column, both from a lateral and a posterior view, to be able to assess the slightest mal-alignment.

The general posture of the patient will reveal a great deal of useful information for the correct diagnosis of his condition. Although there is great variation in the contours of normal healthy people, an experienced doctor can readily ignore these differences and detect any slight variation from these norms. This will suggest where strain will occur in the back of that patient and may, if severe enough, be actually the result of a back condition and thus point towards the final diagnosis.

These first two chapters attempt to show how a normal healthy back functions and this chapter, in particular, seeks to describe and underline the importance of those features of the spinal column that are concerned with the function and treatment of a slipped disc lesion.

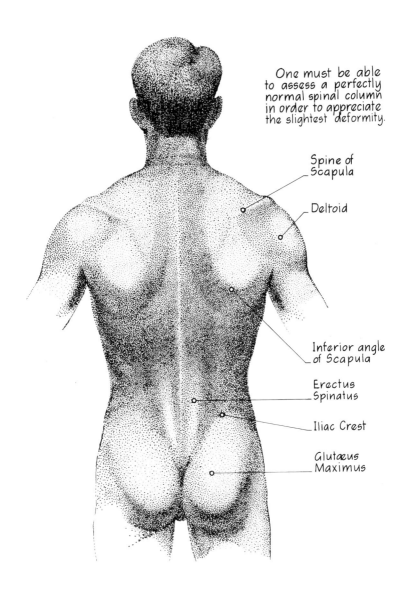

One must be able
to assess a perfectly
normal spinal column
in order to appreciate
the slightest deformity.

Spine of
Scapula

Deltoid

Inferior angle
of Scapula

Erectus
Spinatus

Iliac Crest

Glutæus
Maximus

Diag. 2. Posterior view of the normal back.

16

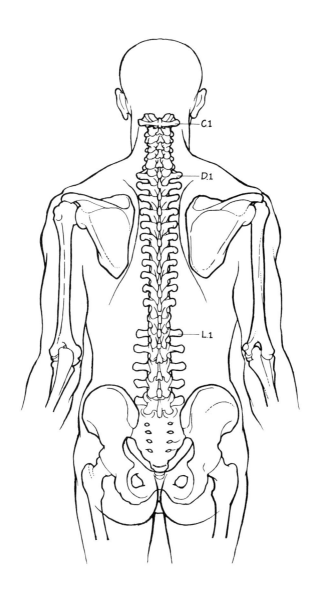

Diag. 3. Posterior view of the spinal column showing its relationship to the body.

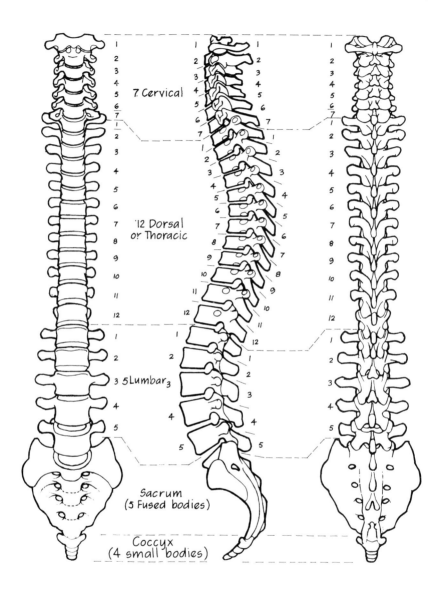

7. Cervical

12 Dorsal
or Thoracic

5 Lumbar

Sacrum
(5 Fused bodies)

Coccyx
(4 small bodies)

Diag. 4. Anterior, lateral and posterior views of the whole spinal column showing the five regions.

18

Composition of the Spinal Column

The spinal column is made up of 33 vertebrae and may be divided into 5 areas or regions:

1) The neck or cervical area, comprising 7 vertebrae.
2) The chest or dorsal (thoracic) area, comprising 12 vertebrae.
3) The lower back or lumbar area, comprising 5 vertebrae.
4) The sacrum, which is a wedge shaped bony mass made up of 5 fused vertebrae.
5) The tail of the spinal column or coccyx made up of 4 small vertebrae.

For convenience, the vertebrae are usually referred to by the first letter of the area to which they belong followed by the number showing the position of that vertebra in its area (numbering from the neck to the tail of the column). For example, the first cervical vertebra in the neck (that is the one closest to the skull) is called C.1; the second dorsal vertebra in the chest area, D.2; the fifth lumbar vertebra in the lower back, L.5; the first sacral vertebra, S.1 and so on.

The Mechanical functions of the Spinal Column

The spinal column performs five main mechanical functions:

1. It forms a canal, or casing, for the safety of the spinal cord and the fine nerve roots which emerge from the cord and extend to the peripheral parts of the body.
2. It is a bony structure, so designed to permit great flexibility, subservient to the motor functions of the whole body.
3. Basically it is a jointed, sustaining rod, maintaining the upright posture and by so doing, it carries the body weight. Movement is present to a moderate degree through the articulation of the facet joints behind, or posteriorly, and through the annular ligament between each two opposing vertebral bodies in front, or anteriorly.
4. It forms a post for the anchorage of the powerful muscles of the trunk, pelvic girdle, the shoulders and the neck.
5. Through the annular ligament, it acts as a cushion or buffer-like spring, thus receiving and distributing an almost constant series of jolts and jars to which our bodies are subjected daily. The facet joints are so aligned as to prevent the collapse of one vertebra on to another, thus avoiding damage to the spinal cord and its nerve roots.

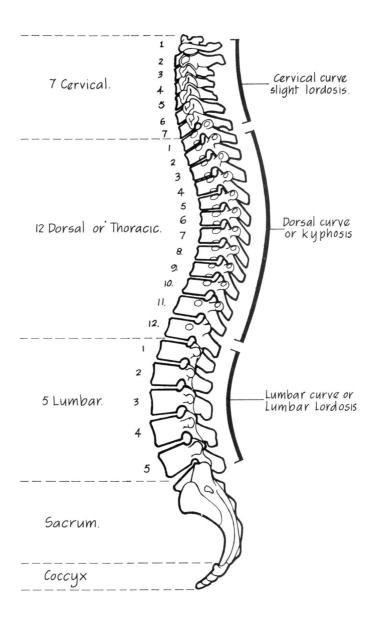

7 Cervical.

1
2
3
4
5
6
7

Cervical curve
slight lordosis.

12 Dorsal or Thoracic.

1
2
3
4
5
6
7
8.
9.
10.
11.
12.

Dorsal curve
or kyphosis

5 Lumbar.

1
2
3
4
5

Lumbar curve or
Lumbar Lordosis

Sacrum.

Coccyx

Diag. 5. Lateral view of the vertebral column showing the normal adult contour.

Any of these mechanical functions of the spinal column, or any combination of them, may fail because of some underlying local or general cause. For example, it can fail to act as a sustaining rod through weakness or the inefficiency of the musculature which supports it.

The Notochord

Part of the spinal column is developed from the notochord which is defined as the primitive axis of the body, a rod shaped mass composed of cells derived from the mesoblast. During foetal development, a fibrous sheath gradually develops around the notochord and as the foetus becomes larger and more complex this sheath requires stiffening for muscular attachments. It is then converted into cartilage and finally into bone. This stiffening would result in loss of mobility if the bony rod were not segmented into separate vertebrae, which articulate with one another. At the same time the nerve cord, (which eventually becomes the spinal cord) runs along the dorsal side of the notochord and becomes protected and made to follow the movements of the backbone by a series of cartilaginous rings which later on become bony. These rings join with the bodies of all the vertebrae.

The disc is considered to be a remnant of this early notochord, from which it is developed, and its repeated absence in dissected cases also suggests this.

Anatomical Considerations of the Spinal Curves

In the foetus the thoracic and sacral curves only are present in the spinal column, but after birth, as the child assumes the erect posture, two secondary curves develop, the cervical and the lumbar. Normally, until puberty, when standing erect, these primary and secondary curves pass almost imperceptibly into one another preserving the balance of the trunk by concavity alternating with convexity. Theories have been advanced that the prevalence of slipped disc lesions is a direct result of man adopting the erect posture and that man, at one time, normally walked on all fours. Personally I do not accept this theory. However, it may well be right and one must wait until sufficient proof has been brought to bear on the subject.

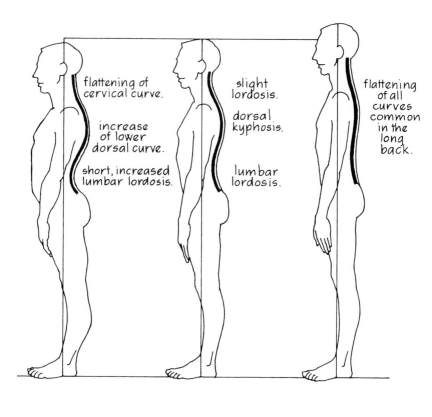

flattening of cervical curve.

increase of lower dorsal curve.

short, increased lumbar lordosis.

slight lordosis.

dorsal kyphosis.

lumbar lordosis.

flattening of all curves common in the long back.

Heavy Muscular Type

Normal

Flat Back

Diag. 6. The adult contour showing normal variations.

22

Lordosis

Curvature of the spinal column with a forward convexity is known as lordosis. The forward curve, or normal lumbar lordosis, which is more pronounced in the female than the male, begins at the middle of the last thoracic vertebra and ends at the anterior surface of the lumbo-sacral joint. The latter point, which in the erect posture, is said to be vertically under the occipital condyles, (the base of the skull) marks the commencement of the sacral concavity — a concavity which faces downwards and forwards, and extends to the tip of the coccyx. Lordosis is also present in the cervical area, affecting the lower 3 cervical joints. It develops when the child holds his head up at the third month, whereas the lumbar curve develops when the child sits up, usually after 6 months.

Kyphosis

Curvature of the spinal column showing a backwards convexity is called kyphosis and is normally present in the thoracic region, but can become exaggerated as a result of a dorsal disc lesion or faulty posture. This frequently develops in the aged.

The presence of normal lordosis and kyphosis varies from individual to individual. The tall and slender anatomical type usually has a relatively long flat back. These people are generally considered to be more prone to the slipped disc condition, but after a close study, taking 500 cases at random, I firmly conclude that this belief has no factual clinical foundation. As long as the muscles are in good tone, the normal long-backed individual suffers no more, nor no less, from disc lesion, than the person with the short back. Those with the long backs do have a moderate degree of flattening of the normal lumbar lordosis and to a lesser degree flattening of the normal thoracic kyphosis. Thus the body is carried backwards by hyperextension in the lumbar region, making a sharp curve at the lumbo-sacral level, and the line of gravity is deflected strongly backwards. It is the muscles of the spinal column that maintain its shape and not the bony articulation.

Alternatively, there is the heavy muscular type of patient, with a wide costal angle, heavy flat and broad vertebrae and a short lumbar region. These patients have an increase in the lumbar lordosis, forming quite a hollow in the lumbar region and mobility of the

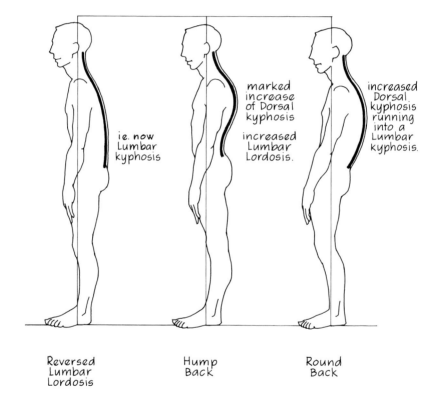

ie. now
Lumbar
kyphosis

marked
increase
of Dorsal
kyphosis

increased
Lumbar
Lordosis.

increased
Dorsal
kyphosis
running
into a
Lumbar
kyphosis.

Reversed
Lumbar
Lordosis

Hump
Back

Round
Back

Diag. 7. Common abnormalities of the adult contour.

24

lumbar area is rather restricted. The kyphosis of the upper trunk, (i.e. the thoracic curve), is recovered by a compensatory lordosis. Thus the line of gravity is a little deflected and the pelvis retains its normal position.

Posture must be defined in terms of the relationship of the line of gravity to the landmarks of the lumbar body and not, as is commonly done, by the relationship of the body parts to each other.

Development of Abnormalities

As adult stature is reached, the constant weight of the trunk increases the sharpness of the lumbo-sacral angle. This weight is borne by the opposing surfaces of the vertebral bodies through the inter-vertebral disc complex anteriorly, and to a lesser extent by the articular processes (facets) posteriorly. In the healthy adult with a normally developed spinal column, the curvatures are such as to allow these surfaces to take the bulk of the downward pressure and the erect posture is maintained by the tone of the musculature, without excessive strain being placed upon the muscles and ligaments of the vertebral column.

If, owing to ill-health or in old age, the tone of the musculature is diminished, the weight causes an exaggeration of the normal curvatures and throws a strain upon the ligaments and articular surfaces. The effect of this is most marked at the lowest part of the trunk where the flexible upper part of L.5 articulates with the rigid extremity of the upper surfaces of the sacrum, that is, at the lumbo-sacral joint. Similarly, if the bony structures of these areas have a congenital weakness, or their strength is diminished by any pathological process, the super-incumbent weight will produce deformities of a nature dependent upon the position and extent of the weakness or lesion. Such congenital weakness of the spinal column may result in adolescent scoliosis (see Chapter IX). The slipped disc condition often also gives rise to abnormal curvatures of the spinal column.

In the slipped disc condition the repeated striking of the disc on the nerve root causes it to become hypersensitive and the muscles supplied by it to go into spasm. If the muscles in spasm are in the posterior aspect of the spinal column it may be pulled backwards causing a flattening of the normal lumbar curve, and it may even force this curve into reverse, giving rise to lumbar kyphosis. The normal curve in the thoracic area is a kyphosis. Thus if the posterior muscles here are affected the increase of kyphosis gives rise to varying degrees of **'Hump Back'** or **'Round Back'** (see also Chapter IX).

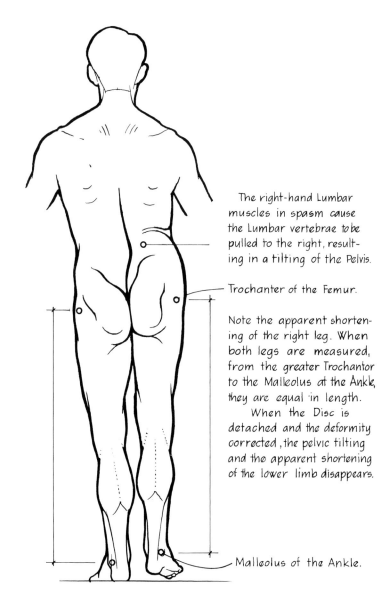

The right-hand Lumbar muscles in spasm cause the Lumbar vertebrae to be pulled to the right, resulting in a tilting of the Pelvis.

Trochanter of the Femur.

Note the apparent shortening of the right leg. When both legs are measured, from the greater Trochantor to the Malleolus at the Ankle, they are equal in length.

When the Disc is detached and the deformity corrected, the pelvic tilting and the apparent shortening of the lower limb disappears.

Malleolus of the Ankle.

Diag. 8. Posterior view of the back showing scoliosis to the right as a result of a slipped disc lesion in the lumbar area.

Scoliosis

If the muscles, that are in spasm due to a disc lesion, are to one side of the spinal column, these lateral muscles, in spasm, will pull the spinal column to the affected side. This may lead to a lateral curvature of the spinal column and is known as 'scoliosis'. It can occur at any level in the spinal column. If it occurs in the cervical region, it is specifically called 'torticollis'. Lateral curvature of the spinal column or scoliosis is most pronounced when it occurs as a result of a disc lesion in the lumbar region and in this case, the scoliosis may persist into the gluteal area. These lumbar muscles are so powerful that, in spasm, they may cause the pelvis to be raised at the affected side. A tilting of the pelvis results, causes an apparent shortening of one of the lower limbs but, after the correct treatment for the slipped disc lesion is given, the spastic muscles will gradually relax and the pelvis will once again assume its normal horizontal position and the legs will appear to be of the same length.

If the lateral muscles are involved at the same time as the muscles in the posterior aspect of the spinal column are affected in the lower back or at the base of the neck, a lumbar or cervical kypho-scoliosis could occur.

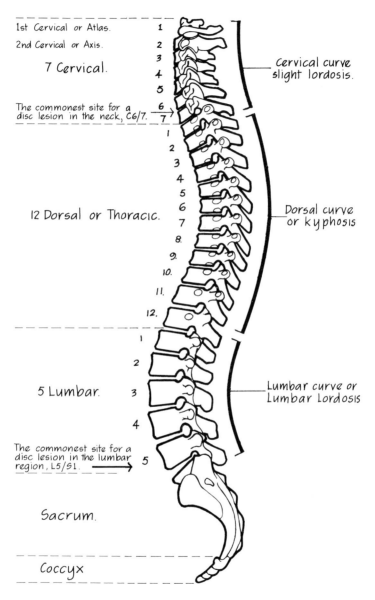

1st Cervical or Atlas.   1

2nd Cervical or Axis.   2

3

7 Cervical.   4

5

The commonest site for a   6
disc lesion in the neck, C6/7.   7

Cervical curve
slight lordosis.

1

2

3

4

5

6

12 Dorsal or Thoracic.   7

8.

9.

10.

11.

12.

Dorsal curve
or kyphosis

1

2

5 Lumbar.   3

4

Lumbar curve or
Lumbar Lordosis

The commonest site for a
disc lesion in the lumbar
region, L5/S1.   5

Sacrum.

Coccyx

Diag. 9. Lateral view of the spinal column showing commonest sites for disc lesions.

28

Commonest Sites for Disc Lesions

The anatomical configuration of the spinal column gives rise to two vulnerable sites in particular and these are the sharp angles of the secondary curves. Thus the majority of disc lesions occur between L.5/S.1, whilst the next most common site in the lumbar region is between L.4/5. Rarely are other areas of the lumbar region affected. In the lowest lumbar region the weight of the whole trunk, bearing down on the sharp angle between L.5/S.1 produces strain at this level that can cause a disc lesion. A contributory factor also may be the wedge shape of the fifth lumbar vertebra for it is deeper anteriorly (in front) than posteriorly (behind). Its features markedly distinguish it from other vertebrae. The annular ligament at its posterior aspect is very thin between L.4/5 and L.5/S.1. The combined qualities of the thin posterior annular ligament and the wedge-like shape of the 5th lumbar make the area at this level the commonest site for disc lesions in the whole spinal column.

In the neck, the disc between cervical 6/7 is most commonly affected. The neck holds the weight of the head during forward flexion, as in such common activities like eating, sleeping, writing, and most of the strain of this is borne by cervical 6/7.

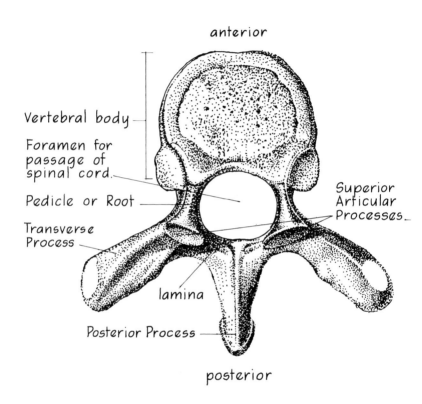

anterior

Vertebral body

Foramen for
passage of
spinal cord.

Pedicle or Root

Transverse
Process

Superior
Articular
Processes.

lamina

Posterior Process

posterior

The Vertebral Arch consists of :-
(i) a pair of Pedicles, and (ii) 7 processes,

ie. 4 Articular (facets),
   (2 superior only are shown)
   2 Transverse, or lateral,
   1 Posterior.

Diag. 10. A complete vertebra from above.

Structure of a Vertebra

A **Vertebra** consists of two essential parts, the front or anterior segment called the body and the rear or posterior segment which is called the vertebral arch. These anterior and posterior processes conjoin to enclose a foramen or space through which passes the spinal cord and their bony configuration serve to protect it. The anterior processes or bodies form a pillar for the support of the head and the trunk, and the column is articulated to allow free movement. Between every pair of vertebrae are two intraverted foramina, one on either side, for the transversion of the spinal nerves and vessels.

The Body is the largest part of the vertebra, and is more or less cylindrical in shape. The upper and lower surfaces are flattened, rough and spongy. Into this rough surface are impaled hyaline cartilaginous plates which have a smooth outer surface against which the disc or nucleus pulposus lies. Around the rim of the body is the strong annular ligament which joins the opposing bodies, encloses the nucleus pulposus and acts as a coil spring to the whole spinal column. In front the body is convex from side to side and concave from above downwards. Its anterior surface presents a few small apertures for the passage of nutrient vessels, whilst on the posterior surface is a single larger aperture, or occasionally more than one, for the exit of the veins from the body of the vertebra.

The vertebral arch consists of a pair of pedicles or roots. It supports seven processes, four articular, two transverse or lateral and one posterior.

The posterior spinous process is directed backwards and downwards from the junction of the laminae and serves for the attachments of the muscles and ligaments.

The transverse or lateral processes project one on either side from the point where the lamina joins the pedicle between the superior and inferior articular processes or facets. They also serve for the attachment of further muscles and ligaments of the spinal column.

The four articular processes or facets spring from the junctions of the pedicles and laminae of each vertebra. Each vertebra has upper and lower pairs of facets, that is two superior and two inferior. The superior processes or facets project upwards and the articular surfaces are directed more or less backwards but anatomical variations do occur quite normally. In fact the ability to touch one's toes is a direct result of the alignment of the facet joints. If they run predominantly in a vertical plane then that person can put his palms on the floor. If the facets articulate in a horizontal plane then the individual,

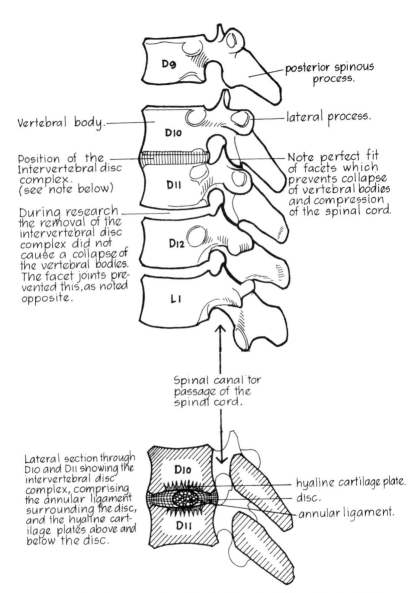

D9

posterior spinous
process.

Vertebral body.

lateral process.

D10

Position of the
Intervertebral disc
complex.
(see note below)

Note perfect fit
of facets which
prevents collapse
of vertebral bodies
and compression
of the spinal cord.

D11

During research
the removal of the
intervertebral disc
complex did not
cause a collapse of
the vertebral bodies.
The facet joints pre-
vented this, as noted
opposite.

D12

L1

Spinal canal for
passage of the
spinal cord.

Lateral section through
D10 and D11 showing the
intervertebral disc
complex, comprising
the annular ligament
surrounding the disc,
and the hyaline cart-
ilage plates above and
below the disc.

D10

hyaline cartilage plate.

disc.

annular ligament.

D11

Diag. 11. Schematic presentations showing the articulation of the facet joints
in a segment of the spinal column and the position of the intervertebral disc
complex.

however fit and healthy, may not be able to reach with his hands beyond his ankles. This is a normal anatomical state and has no pathological significance.

Facet Subluxation

In most of the speciments examined in the anatomy and pathological departments I found the articular facets between L.5 and S.1 to be, predominantly, in the horizontal plane i.e. straight or running in an antero-posterior direction but, at times, these facets beteen L.5/S.1 were, predominantly, in the vertical plane. Variation from the normal was very frequent. This is important clinically if the degree is severe or unilateral, for example one facet being in the horizontal, and the other on the opposite side in the vertical plane. If the greater part of the facet faces backwards, little idea of the condition of the surface of the joint can be obtained from an x-ray, but if the greater part faces inwards then the joint surfaces, with a narrow space between them, can be seen on the x-ray plates, and any irregularity of the surface or displacement of this joint may be detected. In some cases one facet faces backwards and the other inwards. A careful examination of all the x-ray plates of more than 500 patients revealed that 60% had facets in the lumbar regions facing backwards, 10% facing inwards, and 30% had 'mixed' facets, one side facing backwards and the other inwards.

The articular facets of the lumbo sacral joints, in particular, show great variation in their shape as well as the plane of their articular surfaces, and, to a lesser degree, this can occur in any particular joint of the spinal column. The superior articular facets on the majority of sacrums are slightly crescentic but in some cases, the surfaces are quite flat.

During research when a clamp was placed above L.5 and below S.1 and the screw turned, if the facet joint surfaces were lying predominantly horizontally very little movement took place between the vertebral bodies and only a small bulge of the annular ligament occurred. When, however, the same experiment was done when the facet joints were predominantly vertical, there was considerable bulging of the annular ligament and the vertebral bodies were brought close together when the screw was turned. Thus injury in the lumbo sacral area, caused, for example, by falling from a height and landing on one's feet, will increase the forward angulation of this joint L.5/S.1 and if that individual has one facet in the vertical plane, a

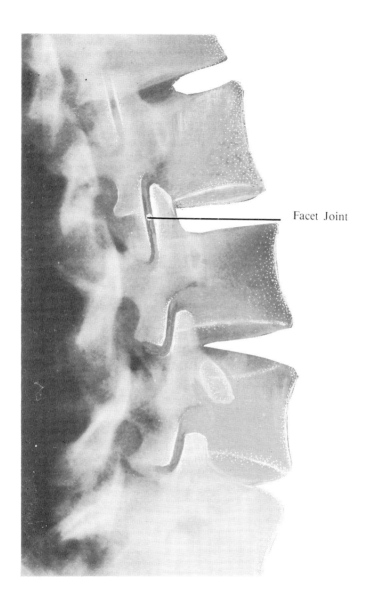

Facet Joint

Diag. 12. Photograph of an X-ray plate showing facet joints articulating in an almost vertical plane.

34

partial dislocation of the joint may occur, i.e. one facet may slip downwards on its opposing facet. In such cases, there is a marked bulging of the annular ligament on the affected side, simulating a slipped disc lesion if the bulging annular ligament strikes a nerve root. The symptoms and treatment are given in Chapter IX, page 149.

In the cervical area the facet joints incline upwards and tend to be more vertical than in the lumbar region. Thus, following a whiplash injury, dislocation of the cervical vertebrae can occur without fracture. Anywhere else in the spinal column a pure dislocation usually cannot occur because of the direction of the facets, and severe injury, in this case, usually causes a fracture dislocation, as the facets must break off before the spinal bodies can move apart.

The facets and the coil spring-like annular ligament are the factors that prevent the vertebral bodies from collapsing onto one another. This permits the slipped disc to be removed without damage to the mechanism of the spinal column.

Spondylolisthesis

I have noted that with asymmetrical development of the articular processes abnormal movements may occur in the spinal column. Obviously the flat type gives stability in one field only, so that any excessive force directed in another plane will strain the ligaments of the joint and, indeed, may cause a subluxation of this joint showing the clinical features of a slipped disc lesion. One significant example

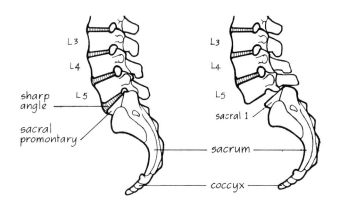

Diag. 13. Spondylolisthesis.

35

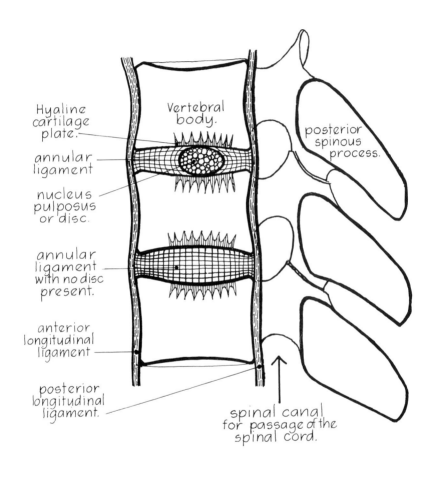

Hyaline
cartilage
plate.

annular
ligament

nucleus
pulposus
or disc.

annular
ligament
with no disc
present.

anterior
longitudinal
ligament

posterior
longitudinal
ligament.

Vertebral
body.

posterior
spinous
process.

spinal canal
for passage of the
spinal cord.

Diag. 14. Section through a segment of the spinal column showing the
position of the intervertebral disc complex.

36

of this is the separation of the neural arch of the 5th lumbar vertebra, together with its inferior articular processes from its normal position and this results in a forward dislocation of the 5th lumbar from the sacrum. This is called **'Spondylolisthesis'.** This, in my opinion, causes the low back pain and the scoliosis that has long defied explanation. This condition can also occur between L.4 and L.5, but very rarely, at a higher level, except as a result of a severe accident.

The Anatomy of the Structures sited between Two Opposing Vertebral Bodies
— The intravertebral disc complex.

The intravertebral disc complex structures form about one quarter of the length of the vertebral column and are largest in the lumbar region. In the cervical and lumbar regions, they are deeper in front than behind and this gives rise to a forward curve in the cervical and lumbar regions. In the thoracic region they are of uniform depth. Throughout the column they are intimately connected with the anterior and posterior longitudinal ligaments, and in the thoracic region, with the anterior costo-central ligaments and the inter-articular ligaments of the heads of most of the ribs. In the cervical region the intervertebral disc complex is seldom present at either lateral aspect of the opposed surfaces of the bodies. In this region there is a synovial space on either side, between the projecting lateral lip of the upper surface of the lower body, and the bevelled lateral margin of the lower surface of the upper body. The opposed surfaces are covered by cartilage and there is an indistinct capsular ligament sometimes surrounding a rudimentary disc.

After the age of 65 or in later life the whole of the intervertebral disc area, particularly the annular ligament, begins to atrophy, becomes thinner, and often gives rise to the bowing of the back in old age with a loss of height which could be on average from 3-7 inches.

Between opposing vertebral bodies are three separate structures or three varieties of tissue and they are so important to this thesis that they must be considered separately.

These are 1. **The Annular Ligament**
2. **Disc** i.e. The Nucleus Pulposus
3. **The Hyaline Cartilage Plates**

37

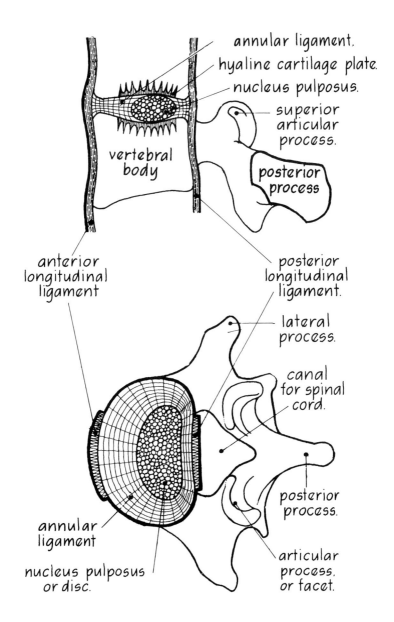

Diag. 15. Longitudinal and transverse section of the intervertebral disc complex in the lumbar region.

1. **The Intervertebral Annular Ligament**

These ligaments are situated between the adjacent surfaces of the bodies of the vertebrae and they constitute the chief bond of union between them. Their outline corresponds to that of the outer rim of the bodies between which they are placed. They are elastic and compressible. Each is composed of a circumferential fibrous part, disposed in the form of superimposed laminae, surrounding a central portion which is soft and pulpy and is, in reality, the so-called 'disc'. The external laminar part forms more than half of the disc complex and is composed of fibrous tissue and fibro-cartilage. In transverse section the laminae are seen to be arranged concentrically around the central disc which they closely embrace and compress. The fibres, of which they are composed, are arranged in parallel bundles which extend obliquely between the adjacent surfaces of the vertebral bodies and are attached to the layer of hyaline cartilage which covers them. The fibres of successive laminae pass obliquely in opposite directions. The outer laminae consist of fibrous tissue but the majority are composed of white fibro-cartilage. In vertical section the outermost laminae are seen to bend outwards, and those around the central disc bend inwards, towards it. This arrangement contributes to the elasticity of the vertebral column. The elasticity of the ligament permits movement of the spinal column to a moderate degree. It acts as a coil-like spring, though displaying more the movement of a ball joint. It also acts as a cushion or 'buffer' between the vertebral bodies enabling the spinal column to withstand the jolts and jars that may occur in everyday activities, competitive sport or even in minor accidents.

It completely encloses the nucleus pulposus and keeps it in position between the vertebral bodies. In research it proved to be extremely tough, able to withstand considerable pressure. When clamps were fixed above and below a pair of opposing bodies and when the screw of the clamp was turned, only bulging, but no trauma or tearing of the ligament occurred. In fact an ordinary scalpel could not pierce it and in order to produce a tear or trauma a robust pathological knife had to be used. This tear, when produced, simulated, as it were, a slipped disc lesion, for it allowed the nucleus pulposus to burst through the ligament with the possibility of striking a nerve root.

In every day life, a similar trauma can occur naturally when the annular ligament at the point of greatest stress caused by the body weight, and a summation of minor injuries, becomes so thin that a sudden movement may cause it to rupture. This tear allows the nucleus pulposus to burst through this thin area of ligament and, if it should strike a nerve root or tract, will produce the painful symptoms associated with the slipped disc lesion condition.

The annular ligament is at its thinnest and weakest in its posterior aspect but a lesion in the ligament here is prevented, except as a result of an extremely rare and serious accident, by the presence of the strong posterior longitudinal ligament. Very, very seldom does a prolapsed disc come into contact with the spinal cord itself because of the protective intervention of this posterior ligament. Thus the most vulnerable and most common site for trauma or injury of the annular ligament is at its postero-lateral aspect and this aspect at each side corresponds with the position of the emergence of the nerve roots from the spinal cord, through the intraverted foramina.

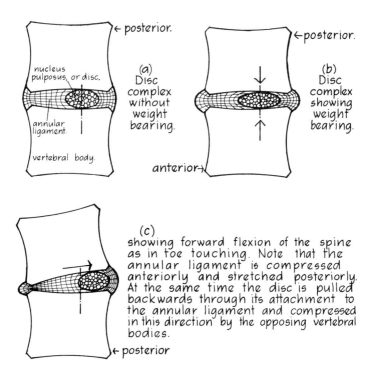

Diag. 16. Schematic view showing the position of the annular ligament in spinal movement.

40

The Disc or Nucleus Pulposus

The disc is firm and elasticated with a jelly-like consistency. In many cases it is semi-fluid, being the myxomatous remains of the notochord from which it is derived. At birth most of us have a small portion of the notochord, i.e. disc or nucleus pulposus, left in situ within the annular ligament that separates two vertebral bodies, but, in other people, the notochord is completely absorbed leaving no disc at all. This absence was demonstrated clearly during research in the Pathology Department.

The disc consists of an elastic pulpy substance and has a lobate arrangement. It is composed of a cellular reticulum supported by a delicate fibrous stroma. The disc is surrounded and compressed on all sides by the annular ligament and is usually under considerable tension when movement of the spinal column occurs, for it takes its shape from that of the annular ligament. This latter, acting as a cushion or shock absorber between each two opposing vertebral bodies and also providing the "spring" to allow movement, is constantly relaxing or compressing to fulfil its function and thus in turn the disc within must experience similar and considerable tension. When the ligament, as a result of over-stress, tears, the disc, i.e. the nucleus pulposus, bursts forth. If the disc bursts through the ligament laterally or anteriorly where there are no nerve tracts the patient suffers no more than a little discomfort or stiffness in the region of the lesion and the symptoms usually pass off in a few days without treatment. However, the prolapsed disc very often protrudes through the postero-lateral aspect where the ligament is weakest and it is in this area that the nerve roots emerge from the spinal cord. The pulposus itself has no chemical or irritant properties but if it should strike a nerve root, the root will become compressed and give rise to great pain. It will usually cause the muscles supplied by this nerve to go into spasm and curvature of the spinal column may take place as a result. If the disc is broken off, as I shall be proposing later in my non-surgical detachment treatment, the disc no longer acts as a foreign body, for, of itself, its substance is non irritant (or toxic) and it will either lie between muscle planes and be absorbed into the bloodstream and eliminated as a waste product; or fall into the region of the cauda equina. Such pieces of disc were often found during dissection.

The disc is not essential to one's anatomy. In the theory, evolved by Schmorl in 1928, he suggested that the disc or nucleus pulposus, may possibly act as a cushion or buffer between each two opposing vertebral bodies, but I, from the results of my research, have been able to demonstrate that it is the annular ligament which is the real cushion or buffer and not the disc or nucleus pulposus. To help to confirm my theory, I was able to demonstrate in the pathology department that many of the specimens who had died of various diseases had no discs at all and yet during their lifetime had had no history of back trouble whatsoever. I thus concluded that the annular ligament can perform its function as spring or buffer in the spinal column quite satisfactorily without the disc. The vertebral bodies do not come together in its absence because of the presence of the annular ligament and that of the articular processes or facets of the opposing vertebrae. However, it must be said the latter do sometimes show abnormal anatomical relationship and this allows these articular facets to slide over one another. This can simulate the clinical picture of a slipped disc lesion and must be separately diagnosed (see Chapter IX). In this case, the opposite vertebral bodies may come close together but, as explained, this is because of the arrangement of the facet joints and not due to the absence of the disc.

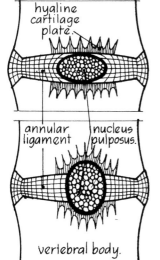

(a) The normal intervertebral disc complex.

(b) Schmorl's Nodes. In this case the nucleus pulposus expands vertically into the vertebral body pushing the cartilagenous plate, above and below, into the cancellous bone of the vertebra.

Diag. 17. Schmorl's nodes.

The Hyaline Cartilage Plates

These are positioned above and below each nucleus. They lie on the spongy cancellous bone or sieve-like surface of the vertebral bodies and are firmly fixed in this position by spicules of cartilage which are embedded into the vertebral body, thus permitting no movement of the plate. The surface of this plate which lies against the disc has a very highly polished surface. A popular misconception is that this plate is the so-called 'disc' because of its resemblance in shape to a disc-like object and because of its polished surface that suggests it could 'slip'. This is not so.

The plates provide the disc with nutrient by diffusion, and the disc remains viable even when protruding through a tear in the annular ligament as long as it receives its nutrient factor through contact with these plates. When the disc is detached from its nutrient supply it quickly starts to atrophy and then causes no adverse symptoms.

Examination of these cartilage plates showed they varied in thickness from a thin layer of hyaline cartilage to about ¼ ″ in depth. Because they are firmly embedded into the vertebral bodies, even in the most severe whiplash injury to the spinal column causing a massive tear in the annular ligament with complete prolapse of the disc no movement occurs in these plates. Only when a severe fracture of a vertebral body occurs is there any movement of these cartilage plates.

If this cartilage is damaged following severe injury the disc may penetrate the vertebral body, and it may also do so in cases of osteoporosis. This penetration of the disc is known as **'Schmorl's Nodes'** or Nucleus Expansion. There are few symptoms except some loss of movement in the segments involved with a degree of pain and discomfort. Positive diagnosis can be made by x-ray and this is, in fact, the only sure way of positively diagnosing it. It usually occurs in the thoracic region and it may be caused by continuous forced flexion of the spinal column and jumping from heights and landing on the feet, particularly in youth. Toe touching exercises should be reduced to a minimum because of this possible danger of damage to these plates. It may also be caused by a congenital weakness in the cartilage plates. During dissection, in many specimens with such imperfect cartilage plates the disc had penetrated the vertebral body and, in a very few pathological specimens, the cartilage plate or plates were absent altogether, thus easily permitting the expansion of the disc into the vertebral body.

43

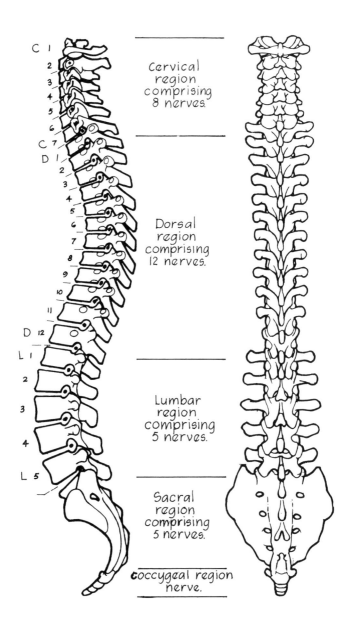

Diag. 18. Lateral and posterior views showing nerves and regions.

44

The Development and Description of the Nervous System with Particular Reference to the Disc Lesion

THE SLIPPED disc condition cannot be fully understood, or treated by my method of non-surgical detachment, without a detailed knowledge of the nervous system, with particular reference to those nerve roots which emerge from the spinal cord. When the disc prolapses as previously explained, through the weakest part of the annular ligament at its postero-lateral aspect it usually strikes a nerve root and it is the position of that particular root which will give rise to the particular symptoms of that disc lesion. Also in the technique for detachment which I shall be advocating and describing I inject one drop of local anaesthetic into that particular nerve root to cause the muscles supplied by it to become flaccid and so enable me to gain access to the disc for its detachment. Thus an intricate knowledge of the nervous system, particularly the nerve tracts, is vital not only before the correct diagnosis can be assured and the proposed treatment undertaken, but also to enable the reader to understand the disc lesion condition fully and assess the viability of the treatment to be recommended.

The Nervous System

The nervous system is the most complicated and highly organised of the various systems which make up the human body. It may be divided into two parts, central and peripheral.

The central nervous system consists of (a) an upper expanded portion, the brain contained within the skull and (b) a lower elongated nearly cylindrical portion, the spinal cord, lodged in the vertebral canal. The two portions are continuous with one another at the level of the upper border of the atlas vertebra (first cervical).

The peripheral nervous system consists of a series of nerves by which the central nervous system is connected to the various tissues of the body. For descriptive purposes, these nerves may be arranged in two groups. 1. cerebro-spinal and 2. sympathetic. The two groups are intimately connected and closely intermingled. The cerebro-spinal nerves are forty-three in number on either side — twelve cerebral attached to the brain and thirty-one spinal attached to the spinal cord. They are associated with the functions of the special and general senses and with the voluntary movements of the body. The sympathetic nerves transmit impulses which bring about constriction of the small arteries and, in association with cerebro-spinal nerves, regulate the movements of the intestines. They are also concerned with the process of secretion. In relation with them are two rows of central ganglia situated one on either side of the middle line in front of the vertebral column. These ganglia are intimately connected to the spinal cord and the spinal nerves and are also joined to each other by vertical strands of nerve fibres so as to constitute a pair of knotted cords. The sympathetic trunks reach from the base of the skull to the coccyx.

The nervous system is built up of nervous and non-nervous tissues.

Spinal Cord

The spinal cord is the elongated, nearly cylindrical, part of the central nervous system which occupies the upper two-thirds of the vertebral canal or spinal column. Its average length in the male is about 45 cm. and in the female from 42-43 cms. Its weight is about 30 gms. It extends from the level of the upper border of the atlas to that of the lower border of the first or upper border of the second lumbar vertebra. Above, it is continuous with the brain. Below, it ends in the conus medullaris from the apex of which a delicate filament descends as far as the first segment of the coccyx.

The position of the spinal cord varies with the movements of the vertebral column, its lower extremity being raised slightly when the column is flexed. It also varies at different periods of life. Up to the third month of the foetal life (before birth) the spinal cord is as long as the vertebral canal, but from this stage onwards the vertebral column elongates more rapidly than the spinal cord. At about the sixth month of foetal life, the cord is at the base of the sacrum whereas at birth it is about level with the third lumbar vertebra. This is an important factor when assessing the exact site of the particular nerve root to be injected because, as a result of this the nerve roots do not correspond exactly with the level of the posterior process of a particular vertebra. This is explained more fully later in this chapter.

The spinal cord does not fill the part of the vertebral canal in which it lies. It is ensheathed by three protective membranes, separated from each other by two concentric spaces. The three membranes are named, from without inwards, the **Dura Mater,** the **Arachnoid** and the **Pia Mater.** Together they are called the Meninges and are the protective membranes of the brain and spinal cord. There is also watery fluid known as the cerebro-spinal fluid which also protects the brain and cord by acting as a fluid cushion.

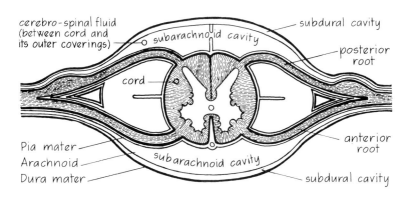

cerebro-spinal fluid (between cord and its outer coverings)

subarachnoid cavity

subdural cavity

posterior root

cord

Pia mater
Arachnoid
Dura mater

subarachnoid cavity

anterior root

subdural cavity

Diag. 19. Transverse section through the spinal cord.

In slipped disc cases where the disc is pressing, for example, on the sciatic nerve root, a cough or sneeze causes the pain in the nerve to be exaggerated. This is due to an increase in cerebro-spinal fluid pressure in the brain transmitting a fluid wave pressure down the cord onto the sensitive area where the disc is pressing on a nerve root. This may cause an onset of sciatica or aggravate a pre-existing sciatic pain. When a disc is striking the brachial plexus in the neck, pain can be similarly exaggerated in the affected nerve tracts, by a sudden cough or sneeze.

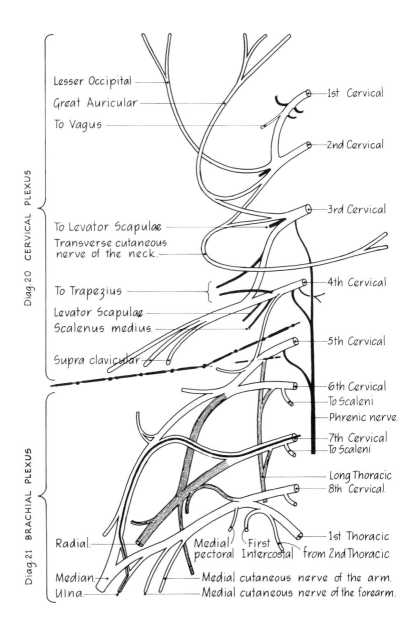

Diags. 20 and 21 Showing the plan of cervical and brachial plexus.

Origin of the Spinal Nerves

There are thirty one pairs of spinal nerves which arise from the sides of the spinal cord. They are arranged in five areas on either side as follows: the cervical, eight in number; the thoracic, twelve; the lumbar, five; the sacral, five and the coccygeal, one. See diag. 18.

1. **The Cervical Region.** This is composed of the cervical plexus and the brachial plexus. The cervical plexus is made up of nerves C.1, 2, 3 and 4. If these nerves are affected by a disc lesion, cervical spasm occurs at this level and, in many cases, a slight scoliosis to the affected side results, plus a migraine-like syndrome, particularly if the disc strikes between the base of the skull and C.1. The brachial plexus is made up of nerves, C.5, 6, 7, 8 and D.1. Two of the largest and most commonly struck nerves of the brachial plexus are the median nerve and the ulnar nerve, in particular. The median nerve passes from the brachial plexus down to the radial side of the elbow, down the forearm on the thenar or thumb side of the hand and supplies the five muscles of the thenar group of the thumb. The ulnar nerve travels along the ulnar aspect of the forearm to the small finger, and supplies the remaining 15 intrinsic muscles of the hand, i.e. the hypothenar eminence.

2. **The Dorsal or Thoracic Region** comprises twelve nerves. This is the least likely area for disc lesions as in this area very little movement occurs in the opposing vertebrae and these vertebrae are further stabilised by the articulation with the ribs. The two most common sites of injury are C.7/D.1 (at the base of the neck) where most movement in this area occurs and a disc lesion here can lead to a brachial neuritis; and secondly at D.12/L.1 where a moderate degree of movement takes place, and a disc lesion here can lead to a lumbago and/or a girdle pain to the lower anterior abdominal wall, giving features of a renal colic or appendicitis if it occurs on the right side. Disc lesions between these two sites are uncommon. However, a disc lesion between D.7/8 can occur and may give rise to girdle pain to the anterior chest wall which may, if it occurs on the left side, simulate a heart attack.

49

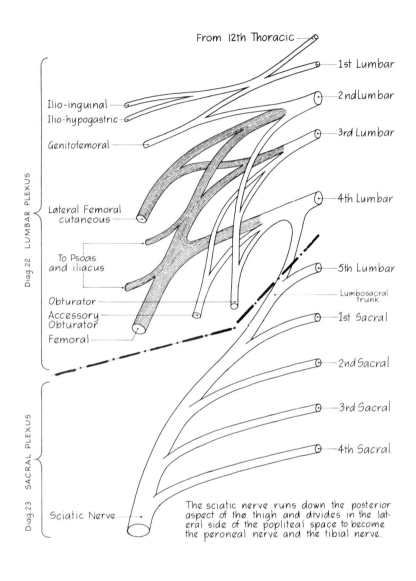

From 12th Thoracic

1st Lumbar

2nd Lumbar

3rd Lumbar

4th Lumbar

5th Lumbar

Lumbosacral trunk.

1st Sacral

2nd Sacral

3rd Sacral

4th Sacral.

Ilio-inguinal
Ilio-hypogastric
Genitofemoral

Lateral Femoral cutaneous

To Psoas and iliacus

Obturator
Accessory Obturator
Femoral

Diag. 22   LUMBAR PLEXUS

Diag 23   SACRAL PLEXUS

Sciatic Nerve

The sciatic nerve runs down the posterior aspect of the thigh and divides in the lateral side of the popliteal space to become the peroneal nerve and the tibial nerve.

Diags. 22 and 23 Showing the plan of lumbar and sacral plexus.

50

3. **The Lumbar Region.** The lumbar plexus is made up of nerves L.1/2/3/4. The fifth lumbar nerve does not form part of the lumbar plexus but a branch from this nerve joins L.4 and thus pain can be referred from L.5 onto L.4 and vice versa, because pain in L.4 by the same tract can be referred along L.5.

If the first lumbar nerve, L.1, is struck by a prolapsed disc, pain will result leading to a moderate lumbago and scoliosis. Pain may radiate along the superior aspect of the pelvic brim, along the inguinal canal giving rise to an **Ilio-Inguinal Neuritis.** If, however, the prolapsed disc strikes the nerves of L.2, 3 or 4 a **femoral neuritis** commonly ensues, giving rise to lumbago, scoliosis and acute pain down the line of the femoral nerve, i.e. from the mid-groin down the anterior aspect of the mid-thigh to just above the knee joint.

If any lumbar nerve is struck the basic clinical symptoms are, as a rule, 1) acute pain in the affected site 2) spasm of all muscles supplied by the nerve struck and 3) a scoliosis due to the muscles in spasm pulling the spinal column towards them.

The Sacral Region

The sacral plexus is made up of L.5, S.1, S.2, S.3, S.4 and S.5. and these nerves join together to become the longest nerve in the body i.e. the sciatic nerve. The commonest site of a disc lesion affecting this plexus is between L.5 and S.1, and gives rise to acute sciatica. The sciatic nerve passes as one large nerve cord into the rear of the pelvis. At this point it lies in a groove in the posterior aspect of the pelvic bone, i.e. the sciatic notch. The nerve then runs down the mid posterior aspect of the thigh to the lateral aspect of the popliteal space. At this point the nerve divides, one large branch emerging at the neck of the fibula, then passing downwards in the lateral aspect of the leg to the lateral malleolus, and the other large branch which is the tibial nerve, passing downwards centrally in the popliteal space, and continuing downwards behind the knee joint to the medial aspect of the os calcis.

The Coccygeal Region

The coccygeal plexus consists of one nerve. Referred pain can occur in this region on one side or the other due to a disc lesion in the lumbar or upper sacral area which leads to a spasm of the erectus spinatus muscle, that is inserted into the coccyx.

51

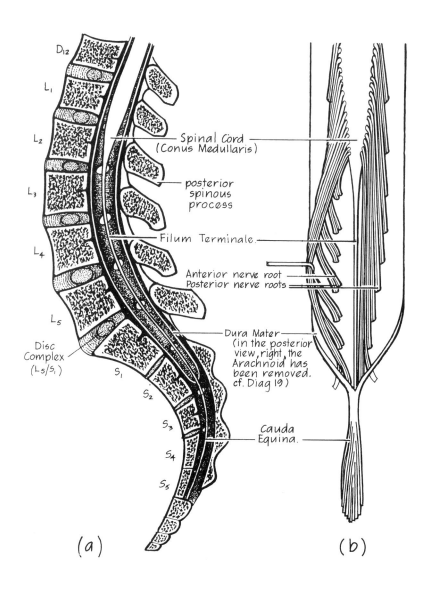

Diag. 24. (a) Lateral and (b) posterior views of the lower part of the spinal cord, showing the filum terminale, and the cauda equina.

The Filum Terminale

The filum terminale is a delicate filament about 20 cm. in length prolonged downwards from the apex of the conus medullaris (i.e. the conoid distal end of the spinal cord). It consists of an upper and a lower part. The upper part, or filum terminale internum, measures about 15 cm. in length and reaches as far as the lower border of the second sacral vertebra. It is contained within the tubular sheath of the dura mater and is surrounded by the nerves forming the cauda equina from which it can be readily distinguished by its bluish-white colour. The lower part, or filum terminale externum, is closely invested by, and is adherent to, the dura mater. It extends downwards from the apex of the tubular sheath and is attached to the back of the first segment of the coccyx. The filum terminale consists mainly of fibrous tissue continuous above with that of the pia mater. Adhering to its outer surface, however, are a few strands of nerve-fibres, which probably represent rudimentary second and third coccygeal nerves. Further, the central canal of the spinal cord extends downwards into it for 5 or 6 cms.

The Spinal Nerves

Each spinal nerve is attached superficially to the cord by two roots, anterior and posterior. Each root consists of several bundles of nerve fibres and at its attachment extends for some distance along the side of the spinal cord. The portion of the cord from which each pair of spinal nerves arises is spoken of as a segment of the cord. Each root is ensheathed by tubular prolongations of the coverings of the cord, namely, the pia mater, arachnoid, and dura mater, in this order from within outwards — and these sheaths ultimately blend with the perineurium (i.e. the connective tissue sheath surrounding a peripheral nerve). The roots are separated from each other by the lateral column of the cord and the ligamentum denticulatum and they pass through separate openings in the theca (or sheath) of the dura mater.

The posterior root is larger than the anterior root and distinguished by the presence of an oval swelling, the spinal ganglion, containing numerous nerve cells. The posterior roots are composed of afferent or sensory fibres which convey impulses from the higher centres of the brain to the periphery. Their fasciculi (or nerve fibres) emerge from the cord in an irregular manner, being spread over an area corresponding in breadth to the caput of the anterior cornu of the grey matter in the interior. These fasciculi (or nerve fibres) enter the cord in a straight line along the course of the postero-lateral sulcus. Each posterior root presents a spinal ganglion and these are for the most part situated in the intervertebral foramina. Immediately beyond each ganglion the anterior and posterior roots unite to form a spinal nerve which is necessarily a mixed nerve in as much as it is composed of Afferent (Sensory) and Efferent (Motor) fibres.

The anterior roots are composed of efferent or motor fibres and their fasiculi (or nerve fibres) emerge from the cord in an irregular manner, being spread over an area corresponding in breadth to the caput of the anterior cornu of the grey matter in the interior.

Diag. 25. Showing the location of the posterior and anterior roots from the spinal cord.

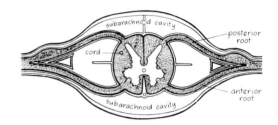

The upper cervical nerve roots are short and pass almost horizontally outwards. The succeeding nerve roots, however, gradually increase in length and incline downwards as they pass outwards. This downward inclination goes on increasing until it becomes almost vertical in the case of the lumbar, sacral and the coccygeal nerves which constitute the cauda equina i.e. tail end of the spinal cord. From this disposition it follows that, in the majority of cases, the superficial origins of the spinal nerves are on a higher level than the intervertebral foramina through which they emerge from the spinal canal.

This is an important factor in the diagnosis of a slipped disc lesion and its treatment by the non-surgical detachment method under local anaesthesia. The surgeon, who is to administer the local anaesthetic to produce a nerve root block, must first know the relationship of the posterior spinous processes of the vertebrae, which he can palpate down the spinal column, to the vertebral bodies between which the nerve roots emerge postero-laterally through the intraverted foramina from the spinal cord. Secondly, he must be able to identify the position of the origins of the nerve roots in relation to the posterior spinous processes. The following explanation is also given in Chapter IV, where the full technique is described. See page 73.

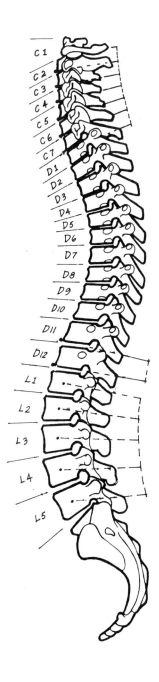

In the case of the cervical and the eleventh and the twelfth thoracic vertebrae, (D11 and D12), the extremities of the spinous processes correspond to the lower margins of the bodies of the respective vertebrae.

In the case of the thoracic vertebrae, from D1 to D10 inclusive, the extremity of each spinous process corresponds to some part of the body immediately below.

See note for cervical above.

In the case of the lumbar vertebrae the extremity of each spinous process corresponds to the centre of the body of its own vertebrae.

Diag. 26. The relationship of the posterior spinous processes of the vertebrae to the vertebral bodies.

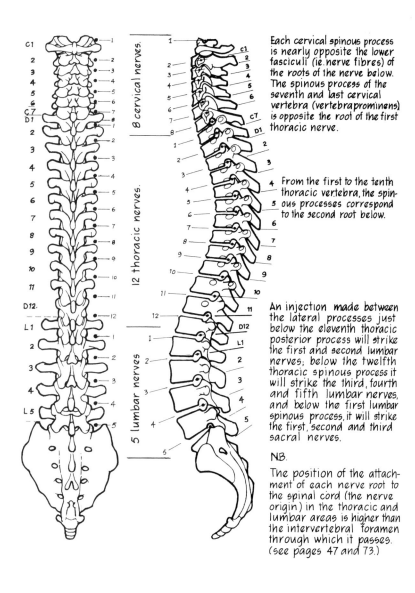

Each cervical spinous process is nearly opposite the lower fasciculi (ie. nerve fibres) of the roots of the nerve below. The spinous process of the seventh and last cervical vertebra (vertebra prominens) is opposite the root of the first thoracic nerve.

From the first to the tenth thoracic vertebra, the spinous processes correspond to the second root below.

An injection made between the lateral processes just below the eleventh thoracic posterior process will strike the first and second lumbar nerves; below the twelfth thoracic spinous process it will strike the third, fourth and fifth lumbar nerves, and below the first lumbar spinous process, it will strike the first, second and third sacral nerves.

N.B.

The position of the attachment of each nerve root to the spinal cord (the nerve origin) in the thoracic and lumbar areas is higher than the intervertebral foramen through which it passes. (see pages 47 and 73.)

Diag. 27. The relationship of the posterior spinous processes to the nerve roots.

The Relationship of the Posterior Spinous Processes of the Vertebrae to the Vertebral Bodies

In the case of the cervical and the eleventh and twelfth thoracic vertebrae the extremities of the spinous processes correspond to the lower margins of the bodies of the respective vertebrae. In the case of the thoracic vertebrae from the first to the tenth inclusive, the extremity of each spinous process corresponds to some part of the body immediately below. In the case of the lumbar vertebrae the extremity of each spinous process corresponds to the centre of the body of its own vertebra.

The Relationship of the Posterior Spinous Processes to the Nerve Roots

Each cervical spinous process is nearly opposite the lower fasciculi (i.e. nerve fibres) of the roots of the nerve below. Similarly, the spinous process of the 7th and last cervical vertebra (vertebraprominens) is opposite the roots of the first thoracic nerve. From the first to the tenth thoracic vertebrae the spinous processes correspond to the second root below. The eleventh thoracic posterior spinous process corresponds to the first and second lumbar nerves. The twelfth thoracic spinous process corresponds to the third, fourth and fifth lumbar nerves. The first lumbar spinous process corresponds to the first, second and third sacral nerves.

Although no trace of transverse segmentation is visible on the surface of the spinal cord, it is convenient to regard it as being built as a series of superimposed spinal segments or neuromeres, each of which has a length equivalent to the extent of attachment of a pair of spinal nerves. Since the extent of attachment of the successive pairs of nerves varies in different parts it follows that the spinal segments are of varying lengths; thus, in the cervical region they average 13 mm: in the mid thoracic region 26mm., while in the lumbar and sacral regions they diminish rapidly from 15 mm. at the level of the first pair of lumbar nerves to 4 mm. opposite the attachments of the lower sacral nerves.

57

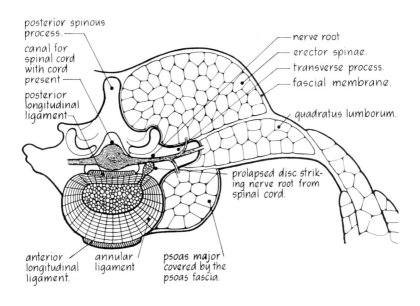

posterior spinous process.

canal for spinal cord with cord present

posterior longitudinal ligament

nerve root

erector spinae.

transverse process.

fascial membrane.

quadratus lumborum.

prolapsed disc striking nerve root from spinal cord.

anterior longitudinal ligament.

annular ligament

psoas major covered by the psoas fascia.

Diag. 28. Section through spinal column showing prolapsed disc striking a nerve root.

CHAPTER III

What is a Slipped Disc?

THE PRECEDING chapters have explained in some detail the nature and function of the disc. However, for those readers who have avoided reading these rather anatomical descriptions and also in order to give a simple and clear basis for the promotion of my method of treatment, a summary of these facts will perhaps be in order here.

What is a Disc?

The disc is a small jelly-like mass enclosed by the annular ligament and sited between each two opposing vertebral bodies from the base of the skull to the top or superior aspect of the sacrum.

The disc is made up of a gelatinous or myxomatous tissue and is a remnant of the notochord from which part of the spinal column is developed. Most of the notochord is absorbed just before birth but a remnant of this pulpy or jelly-like mass normally remains and we refer to it as the nucleus pulposus or disc. This description immediately presents a different picture in the mind from that associated with a disc (or a disc like object) in the minds of many patients. Because of its jelly-like quality it cannot 'slip' from between the vertebrae and be 'put back' as is commonly imagined. The pulpy mass would merely disintegrate if pressure was exerted on it in order to push it back into its position within the annular ligament. The clicks that, during manipulation do occur, may suggest to the patient that the disc is being 'put back' but they cannot be made by the movement of a pulpy or jelly-like mass. They are, in fact, simply due to the facet joints of the vertebrae passing over one another.

The disc, or nucleus pulposus, is enclosed and held in position between the vertebral bodies by the tough cartilaginous annular ligament, and it is the elasticity of this ligament that permits movement of the spinal column to a moderate degree. It acts not only as a 'spring' in the spinal column, but also as a cushion or buffer between the vertebral bodies to enable the spinal column to withstand the jars and jolts to which it is subjected in everyday life.

The articulation, or movement, of the spinal column also depends on small joints called facet joints. These are arranged in pairs, two arising from the upper part of each vertebra and two from the lower part. Each pair articulates with the pair of facets on the vertebra immediately below itself. Between every pair of vertebrae are two small passages or intraverted foramina to allow for the passage of the spinal nerves to their attachment with the cord.

Above and below each disc or nucleus pulposus are positioned cartilaginous plates firmly embedded on to the surface of the vertebral bodies. These are called the hyaline cartilage plates. The surfaces of these plates which lie against the disc are highly polished and this may have been responsible for the mistaken idea that the 'disc' itself is a 'disc-like' object that could 'slip' from between the vertebral bodies. The plates, in fact, provide nutrient to the disc, which remains viable as long as it remains in contact with them. When the disc is detached from this nutrient supply, it quickly atrophies, and in time, will be completely absorbed and disappear.

What Causes a Disc to 'Slip'?

As the disc is firmly held in position by the stout, concentric rings of the annular ligament, it follows that, only when a tear occurs in this ligament, can a disc prolapse, or burst through this damaged ligament. Thus injury, or trauma, plays an important part in all disc lesion cases. This injury may be caused by a simple incident, like that of a motor car accident in which whiplash injury is sustained and a sudden tear in the annular ligament may develop. On the other hand, there could be a summation of minor injuries to this ligament, ranging over a long period of time, that leads to a gradual thinning of it. In these circumstances the ligament may become so thin that a very simple sudden movement, even a cough or a sneeze, will exert sufficient pressure to allow the disc to burst its way through the remaining fibres and produce the symptoms of a slipped disc lesion. As one gets older, the annular ligament often degenerates and becomes less flexible and slightly more brittle, so that even a minor accident: a slip or a fall to the ground — even a sudden jerk — may cause a tear in it.

As mentioned earlier, the two most common sites for the slipped disc lesions in the spinal column are in the neck between C.6/7 and in the lumbar region between L.5/S.1. The curvature of the spinal column is increased at these two points and the weight of the head in the first case, and the weight of the trunk in the second, exert tremendous strain on the annular ligament, especially at its posterior aspect, where the angulation is most acute. This is the part nearest to the spinal cord, and here the intervention of the posterior longitudinal ligament prevents the prolapsed disc striking the spinal cord. The weakest part of the annular ligament, therefore, is at its latero-posterior aspect which corresponds almost exactly to the position of the intraverted foramina through which the spinal nerves emerge from the spinal cord. Thus if the disc prolapses through this part of the annular ligament it quite usually strikes a nerve root, and it is this which gives rise to the crippling pain of a slipped disc. The pain will follow the line of the tract of the nerve affected and will persist as long as the disc continues to strike that nerve root. It may cause all the muscles supplied by this nerve to go into spasm and if the spasm is severe enough cause distortion of the column to take place.

If, however, the protruding disc does not strike a nerve root, pain and some muscle spasm in the affected area will result. This will eventually pass away, though possibly leave a moderate degree of residual stiffness. Occasionally, the prolapsed disc may be in such a position that it does not strike the nerve root continuously and this will produce intense, but intermittent, pain in the area affected.

The Symptoms of a Slipped Disc

The symptoms experienced will depend on the site of the disc lesion. Once a disc has burst its way through the annular ligament, it then acts like a foreign body. Persistent and severe pain is the commonest symptom and this is always due to mechanical pressure of the disc on a nerve root. The exact symptoms will depend on the nerve which is being compressed or struck. For example, in the lumbar region, if a branch of the sciatic nerve is struck, this will give rise to pain referred along the whole length of that nerve and it may extend, in general terms, from the lower back, into the buttocks, down the leg, even sometimes extending as far as the foot (see Chapter V). In the cervical region, if the disc strikes a portion of the brachial plexus, pain may be referred down all, or a branch, of this plexus extending from the shoulder, down the arm on the affected side even at times, as far as the hand. (see Chapter VI). In the dorsal region, the slipped disc will give rise to pain in the affected area and quite commonly pain radiating between the ribs to the anterior chest wall (see Chapter VII).

Again if a disc strikes a nerve root, whether it be in the cervical, dorsal or lumbar region, all muscles supplied by this nerve will go into spasm and pull the spinal column towards them giving rise to a lateral curve of the spinal column or scoliosis. When it occurs in the cervical region, it is often specifically called "torticollis". If the muscles in the anterior aspect of the spinal column are affected they too can go into spasm and pull the spinal column at that level forwards, giving rise to an increase of cervical or lumbar lordosis, i.e. increased hollowing of the base of neck or lower back. If however, the muscles are in spasm in the posterior aspect of the neck or lumbar region, flattening of the cervical or lumbar curves will result. If the dorsal part of the column is affected the muscles in spasm will usually pull the spinal column backwards giving rise to an increase in the normal curve of the chest or dorsal kyphosis.

Conventional Treatment

As already indicated, the cause of pain in a slipped disc lesion is the direct result of mechanical pressure of the disc or nucleus pulposus protruding through the torn annular ligament and pressing on a nerve root. Thus the permanent way of eradicating the pain would be the complete detachment of the offending disc away from the nerve root which is being struck.

Various methods of treatment are practised which include traction, plaster of paris casts, surgical corsets, acupuncture and a variety of forms of manipulation. These, and others, are described in more detail in Chapter VIII. They may, at times, afford some relief, but do not tackle the root cause of the problem. These methods are for the most part simply treating symptoms and very seldom effect a permanent cure.

Surgery is another form of treatment often carried out and this, admittedly, removes the disc from the affected nerve in order to prevent any re-occurrence of the pain of the disc lesion condition. In this operation the disc is gouged out completely through the tear in the annular ligament. It must be understood that this is major surgery and not to be undertaken lightly. Unfortunately, also, the results in most cases leave much to be desired. For example, laminectomy, the cutting of the vertebrae at the affected site to gain access for the operation, may cause weakening of the spinal column at this site. Also during this operation damage to a nerve root or in rare cases, to the spinal cord itself, may occur (see also Chapter VIII).

I have performed operations on slipped discs many times and the results following this type of surgery, in my opinion, are not good, regardless of the surgeon who carries them out. These results were so variable that I decided to carry out some research in order to evolve a safer, and perhaps more reliable, method of treating a slipped disc. The essential result of my researches was to produce a method of treatment whereby one could detach the offending disc without the use of surgery with all its attendant risks.

It was also clear to me that in order to understand fully exactly what the disc was and the true part it played, that a detailed re-examination of the anatomy of the whole of the spinal column was absolutely essential.

Research into the Slipped Disc Condition

The Function of the Disc

Prior to the late 1920's, and even into the early thirties, the nucleus pulposus or disc was being operated upon by neuro-surgeons in the belief that a simple tumour was being removed. However, it soon became accepted that this benign tumour was nothing more than the nucleus pulposus or disc.

It was (and often still is) generally considered that the disc acts as a cushion or buffer throughout the spinal column sited as it is between each two opposing vertebral bodies.

In 1928, a German Pathologist called Schmorl, wrote a brilliant paper, in particular giving a detailed anatomical description of the nucleus pulposus or disc. In this paper he referred to the possible function of the disc. He claimed in theory that the disc acted as a cushion between the bodies of the vertebrae; he did not claim that this was fact, but only suggested theoretically that this was its function. This was nevertheless widely accepted.

However, in my opinion, it is the annular ligament that acts as a cushion or buffer throughout the whole spinal column and not the disc, which, in theory, Schmorl suggested. This strong compressible ligament made up of rings of fibro-cartilage and completely surrounding the disc acts like a coil spring between opposing vertebral bodies. My conclusion is based on the evidence of my research, carried out over a period of ten years in Glasgow.

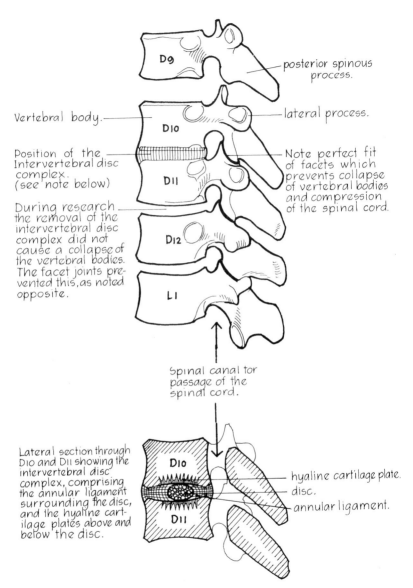

Diag. 29. Schematic presentations showing articulation of the facet joints in a segment of the spinal column and the position of the intervertebral disc complex.

64

My Research

My initial investigation was carried out in the anatomy department of Glasgow University, but I soon concluded that these specimens were dry and distorted and therefore of comparatively little use. I then assessed fresh specimens in the Pathology Department. I found that these gave a far clearer picture of the detailed anatomy of the whole spinal column, all the structures within, and those surrounding it. A clear knowledge of this anatomy is absolutely essential in the assessment and treatment of the slipped disc lesion.

During my research in the Pathology Department I carried out many dissections of the spinal column particularly the area between the vertebral bodies. I noted that quite frequently the spinal discs were not present. These cases had died of various conditions but I took a careful history of these individuals from close relatives and found that 90% had had no history of back trouble. This confirmed my theory that the disc is not an essential part of one's anatomy, and that the annular ligament which surrounds it, is itself the spinal buffer or cushion. Thus the spinal column appears to function perfectly well when the disc is detached. As long as the annular ligament is present there will be no narrowing of the space between opposing vertebral bodies, and thus supported by this ligament, they will not collapse one on the other. Further support preventing collapse is afforded by the presence of the facet joints of the vertebrae.

The anatomy of these facet joints has been described in Chapter I, together with a careful examination of the variations of these joints, which I found in the Pathology Department. I have also described the techniques I adopted during this research in order to show how important these variations are clinically. In the same specimen, for example, I found the articulation of these joints might be in the vertical plane on one side, and in the horizontal plane on the opposite side. If the joints articulate in the vertical plane, there is much more likelihood of these facet joints becoming subluxated when severe downward pressure is exerted on that portion of spinal column. The annular ligament is most vulnerable in these cases and a tear may easily occur with the consequent extrusion of the gelatinous mass of disc. See also diagram 12.

From these two discoveries evolved the basis of my method of treating a slipped spinal disc lesion.

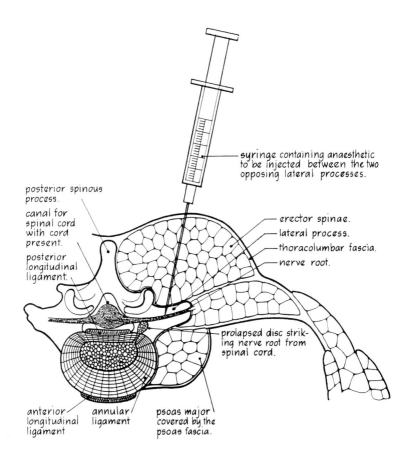

syringe containing anaesthetic
to be injected between the two
opposing lateral processes.

posterior spinous
process.

canal for
spinal cord
with cord
present.

posterior
longitudinal
ligament.

erector spinae.

lateral process.

thoracolumbar fascia.

nerve root.

prolapsed disc strik-
ing nerve root from
spinal cord.

anterior
longitudinal
ligament

annular
ligament

psoas major
covered by the
psoas fascia.

Diag. 30. The injection of local anaesthesia into the affected nerve root to
achieve 'Nerve Root Block'.

66

CHAPTER IV

My Method of Treatment:
The Non-Surgical Detachment of a Slipped Disc Under Local Anaesthesia
i.e. 'Nerve Root Block'

THE ONLY permanent way of curing a slipped disc is to detach the disc which is protruding through the tear in the annular ligament and pressing on a nerve root. The disadvantages of surgery have been described and, with these in mind, I resolved to devise a way of detaching the disc but without the use of surgery.

During the hours spent dissecting specimens in the Pathology Laboratory, I explored in every detail the intricate mechanism of the spinal column and realised that, in order to treat a patient, I could work 'blind', as it were, with my fingers to detach the disc by pressing it against the sharp cutting edges of the torn annular ligament. I also soon realised that, in order to gain access to the site of the disc during the treatment of a patient, the muscles in spasm, because of the compression of the nerve root, must be made to relax. This could be done simply by the injection of a local anaesthetic into the nerve root affected. With the patient's muscles, previously in spasm, now completely flaccid, the spinal column could be flexed to an appreciable degree to allow access for my thumb to the site of the slipped disc. I could then press directly down on to the protruding disc and detach it, cutting it against the sharp edges of the torn annular ligament.

This process, developed from these years in research in the pathological laboratory, I call the non-surgical detachment of a slipped disc under local anaesthesia or nerve root block. It is the essential and unique part of the treatment, for it provides a permanent cure for the slipped disc condition and yet involves none of the attendant risks of surgery.

The patient is asked to keep mobile after this treatment and, in fact, to adopt a training programme prescribed by me and varying according to the position of the disc lesion. This gentle activity will encourage more disc to protrude through the tear and thus at each subsequent treatment (normally 3 or 4 in all) all the disc will eventually be detached.

Once the disc has been detached, the muscles supplied by the affected nerve will gradually relax. However, depending on the length of time that the condition has been allowed to remain untreated, some deformity of the spinal column may have resulted. The correction of such deformity is a further part of my treatment.

My method of treatment for the purposes of giving a clear explanation, may be divided basically into four different aspects.

1. The diagnosis.
2. The non-surgical detachment of the disc under local anaesthesia.
3. Manipulation of the spinal column.
4. The routine training programme of exercises.

1. **The Diagnosis**

Diagnosis plays a vital role in the treatment of a patient and great care and time must be taken to obtain a sure and positive diagnosis for, unless this is correct, the treatment prescribed will be incorrect and worthless. Diagnosis must be thorough and systematic, following a similar pattern in each case. I have set down, in general terms, the main points of diagnosis in the order I consider them during each consultation.

Patient's History When a patient comes for consultation, after the routine details of name, age and address, etc. have been noted, I ask that patient about the pain he is at present suffering and when it began. Then I ask when the first such attack was experienced and gradually build up the history of the whole condition from the first attack through to this present one, noting the duration and severity of each attack.

I enquire what previous treatment has been given; whether x-rays were taken; and, if a disc lesion is suspected, whether any manipulation has been carried out, and by whom.

Neurological Examination Next, I conduct a routine neurological examination, testing the eyes for

1. Equality of pupils
2. Reaction to light and accommodation
3. Presence or absence of nystagmus

and I also check the deep reflexes in the upper and lower limbs.

If these reflexes show too lively a reaction, a more thorough neurological examination is undertaken to eliminate the possibility of multiple sclerosis or similar condition. The presence or absence of the ankle reflex will denote the position of a possible disc lesion in the lumbar region and is a very important and useful diagnostic guide. If this reflex is absent on the affected side then a disc lesion at L.5/S.1, striking the sciatic nerve, is usually the cause.

Inspection For further examination the patient usually stands erect with his back towards me, with the painful area uncovered. Inspection reveals only little information as to the exact area of sensitivity, but careful observation of the posture of the patient and the assessment of any deviation from the correct alignment of the spinal column yields a great deal of information as to the position of a possible disc lesion. Disc lesions are nearly always accompanied by some deviation of the normal alignment of the spinal column: an increase or reduction of the normal lordosis or kyphosis or the presence of scoliosis.

Palpation (or examination by touching) is carried out next and should be done systematically, always considering the exact anatomical structures being palpated. The patient can always tell, or show, the examiner the exact and most tender area of pain and the natural, but illogical, reaction to put a finger on the spot indicated, must be resisted. To do so would increase the pain and create further muscle spasm, thus obscuring the exact location of pain and increasing the difficulties of palpation. It is essential to palpate first those regions which are least apt to give rise to pain, moving inwards at the end of the examination to the most tender spot where the muscles will feel quite hard and in real spasm. Localised tenderness anywhere, as a rule, indicates a lesion in that particular region and this is true of the spinal column as well as any part of the body. In fact, tenderness is even more important in the case of the spinal column, because the structures involved are so deep-seated that any failure of them rarely gives rise to any visible surface change.

The extent of the area of pain and the path it follows (either during this, the patient's present attack or from his description of previous ones) are very significant, for the patient, often unknowingly, will show that the pain follows quite accurately the tract of a nerve and this, in the case of a disc lesion, shows fairly positively which nerve is being affected by the disc and thus indicates the position of the disc lesion.

Differential Diagnosis Diagnosis must be correct and positive. Many conditions have overlapping symptoms and the consultant must systematically consider all possible conditions that would accord with the symptoms being presented, before he eventually comes to a firm conclusion. In the next chapter a detailed description of the differential diagnosis of pain in the lumbar region has been given as an example in order to show the range and importance of this part of the consultation.

This complete pattern of diagnosis is followed, in general, with most patients but is not described in detail again in the chapters concerning cervical or dorsal disc lesion to avoid needless repetition.

X-Ray

If there is any doubt in my mind as to the exact cause of the patient's symptoms I ask for an x-ray to be taken and insist that the plates be taken with the patient in the erect posture, because if taken in the supine posture, distortion of the column will occur. The value of x-ray for the diagnosis of a disc lesion is, actually, rather doubtful, as the disc or nucleus pulposus is not opaque and thus will not show up on the x-ray film. To ensure that a disc lesion does show up, a radio opaque medium, such as myodil, may be injected into the cerebro-spinal fluid. A filling defect will then be visible at the site of the disc protrusion. The disadvantage of this method, however, is that the opaque medium remains in the cerebro-spinal fluid and very often causes varying degrees of headache, which may be chronic. Recently newer soluble media have been developed and these are mostly absorbed eventually. However, this still must be regarded as an unwelcome form of diagnosis, for x-rays themselves are harmful. Usually, the diagnosis of a disc lesion is a quite straightforward clinical diagnosis and the x-ray is only necessary when there is the possibility of a sinister condition of the spinal column. It is invaluable to eliminate the possible presence of a primary or secondary tumour when the diagnosis of a disc lesion is not absolutely certain.

If the positive diagnosis is that of a slipped disc lesion, the detailed symptoms and examination will have revealed the exact position of the disc lesion which, of course, varies from patient to patient, and at this stage the site can be marked with a red pencil. Each condition, its diagnosis and appropriate treatment, is described in detail in the following chapters, but the non-surgical detachment of the disc follows a similar pattern for each area affected. Thus I shall describe it in general terms here and again in specific detail in Chapter V, which describes the treatment for lumbar disc lesions, and thereafter only refer to it to avoid further repetition.

The Injection of Local Anaesthesia into the Affected Nerve Root

The first stage of the treatment is to inject the local anaesthetic into the nerve root on which the prolapsed disc is pressing. The identification of the nerve root involved and the knowledge of the exact position of each vertebral body and the disc complex that separates them is vital before the injection can be made. Chapters I and II give a detailed description of the spinal column and the nervous system but, because this information is so important at this stage of the treatment, a brief explanation is necessary here.

The syringe containing the local anaesthetic is to be guided between the lateral processes of the vertebrae in order to inject into the affected nerve root. The two essential segments that form the vertebrae do not lie in an exact horizontal plane down the length of the spinal column. Thus the posterior processes i.e. the prominences that can be felt down the centre of the back, do not line up directly horizontally with their respective vertebral bodies. These vertebral bodies form the pillar of the column and between each two opposing bodies lies the disc enclosed by the annular ligament. A knowledge of the relationship of the posterior spinous processes (or prominences) to the vertebral bodies is important and may be described as follows:

In the case of the cervical and the eleventh and twelfth dorsal thoracic vertebrae, the extremities of the posterior spinous processes correspond to the lower margins of the bodies of the respective vertebrae.

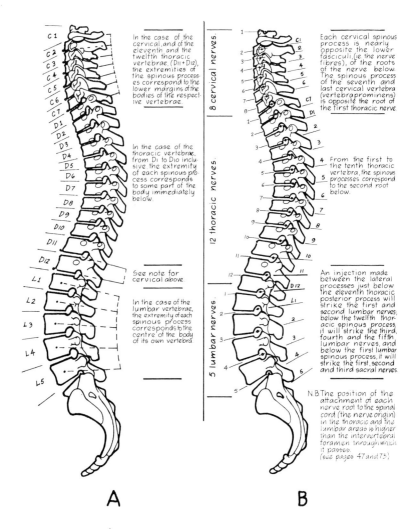

A

In the case of the cervical, and of the eleventh and the twelfth thoracic vertebrae, (D11 + D12), the extremities of the spinous processes correspond to the lower margins of the bodies of the respective vertebrae.

In the case of the thoracic vertebrae, from D1 to D10 inclusive the extremity of each spinous process corresponds to some part of the body immediately below.

See note for cervical above.

In the case of the lumbar vertebrae, the extremity of each spinous process corresponds to the centre of the body of its own vertebra.

8 cervical nerves

12 thoracic nerves

5 lumbar nerves

B

Each cervical spinous process is nearly opposite the lower fasciculi, (ie. the nerve fibres), of the roots of the nerve below. The spinous process of the seventh and last cervical vertebra (vertebraprominens) is opposite the root of the first thoracic nerve.

From the first to the tenth thoracic vertebra, the spinous processes correspond to the second root below.

An injection made between the lateral processes just below the eleventh thoracic posterior process will strike the first and second lumbar nerves; below the twelfth thoracic spinous process, it will strike the third, fourth and the fifth lumbar nerves, and below the first lumbar spinous process, it will strike the first, second and third sacral nerves.

N.B. The position of the attachment of each nerve root to the spinal cord (the nerve origin) in the thoracic and the lumbar areas is higher than the intervertebral foramen through which it passes.
(see pages 47 and 73)

Diag. 31. The relationship of (A) the posterior spinous processes to the vertebral bodies (cf Diag. 26) and (B) the posterior spinous processes to the nerve roots (cf Diag. 27).

72

In the case of the dorsal or thoracic vertebrae from the first to the tenth inclusive, the extremity of each posterior spinous process corresponds to some part of the body immediately below.

In the case of the lumbar vertebrae, the extremity of each posterior spinous process corresponds to the centre of the body of its own vertebra.

Most important of all is the identification of the affected nerve root. The spinal nerve roots arise between each pair of vertebrae, one on either side. However, each pair of nerve roots does not correspond with the exact position of the posterior spinous process (or prominence) of the particular vertebra. This is a result of the relative inequality in the rate of growth of the spinal cord and the spinal column during the development of the foetus (see Chapter II). In the early embryo, the spinal nerves pass transversely from the spinal cord through their respective intervertebral passages or foramina. However, after the third month of foetal life the vertebral column begins to elongate more rapidly than the spinal cord and the nerve roots become longer and more oblique in direction, especially in the lumbar, sacral and coccygeal regions.

Thus the upper cervical nerve roots are short and pass almost horizontally outwards but the succeeding nerve roots gradually increase in length and incline downwards as they pass outwards. This downward inclination goes on increasing until it becomes almost vertical in the lumbar, sacral and coccygeal nerves. Therefore the origins of the spinal nerves, are, in most cases, on a higher level than the intervertebral passages or foramina through which they emerge from the spinal canal. The position of each nerve origin in relation to the corresponding posterior spinous process or prominence can be described as follows (See also page 54):

Each cervical posterior spinous process or prominence is nearly opposite the lower fasciculi (i.e. nerve fibres) of the roots of the nerve below.

The posterior spinous process or prominence of the seventh cervical vertebra is opposite the roots of the first thoracic nerve.

From the first to the tenth thoracic vertebrae the spinous posterior processes or prominences correspond to the second root below.

An injection made between the lateral processes just below the eleventh thoracic spinous process will strike the first and second lumbar nerves; below the twelve spinous process it will strike the third, fourth and fifth lumbar nerves and below the first lumbar spinous process it will strike the first, second and third sacral nerves.

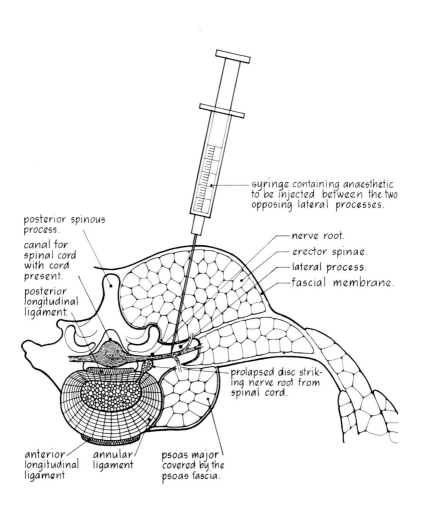

syringe containing anaesthetic
to be injected between the two
opposing lateral processes.

posterior spinous
process.

canal for
spinal cord
with cord
present.

posterior
longitudinal
ligament.

nerve root.

erector spinae.

lateral process.

fascial membrane.

prolapsed disc strik-
ing nerve root from
spinal cord.

anterior
longitudinal
ligament

annular
ligament

psoas major
covered by the
psoas fascia.

Diag. 32. The injection of local anaesthesia into the affected nerve root to achieve 'Nerve Root Block'.

74

2. The Non-Surgical Detachment of the Disc under Local Anaesthesia

In preparation for the injection of the local anaesthetic the patient stands with his back towards me, with the site of the disc lesion uncovered, I check again for the area of the greatest spasticity in the muscle groups on the affected side and this spasticity usually lies under the mark I have already made in red pencil. The area to be injected is carefully cleaned with surgical spirit.

A sterile syringe is prepared and charged with local anaesthesia ready to be injected straight through the muscle groups to a point between the lateral processes of the vertebrae of the spinal column. In order to open up this space, I place a hand on the shoulder of the unaffected side of the body pulling it slowly and gently downwards. I then inject the local anaesthetic into the appropriate nerve root (or into the nerve tract as near as is practicable to its emergence through the outer aspect of the foramen of the vertebra. Injection into the actual nerve root itself may involve some risk of danger to the spinal cord, unless expertly and accurately carried out by an experienced neuro-surgeon and, in practice, provides little more benefit for this particular form of treatment). As soon as the needle touches this nerve root (or tract at the optimum point), the muscles affected by the disc lesion will twitch and this twitching confirms that the needle is in the correct position for the injection of local anaesthetic. It will be noted that the affected muscles which were in spasm, will become flaccid almost immediately, which allows me now to press my thumb firmly through these soft muscles reaching the area between the opposing lateral processes and to come firmly in contact, as it were, with the prolapsed disc. I then press from above downwards on to the sharp cutting edge of the torn annular ligament, and thus the portion of disc protruding through the tear in the annular ligament is detached on the first visit. As I instruct my patients to keep mobile, I usually find on the next visit, another portion of the disc has protruded and this is detached in the same way as the first.

A portion of detached disc may now lie in the muscles planes for some time close to the area of detachment but, once severed from its nutrient supply between the vertebral bodies, it then shrinks, atrophies and is absorbed. It eventually passes out of the body in the urine or faecal matter. In some cases, the detached disc will drop to the bottom of the spinal canal, where it again atrophies and is absorbed. During my research, it was a common finding to locate a portion of disc in the muscle planes and also many pieces of disc in varying degress of atrophy were found at the lower end of the spinal canal i.e. in the region of the cauda equina.

3. Manipulation of the Spinal Column

Manipulation of the spinal column has been practised over many years by the medical profession. Within recent times it has been undertaken by osteopaths, chiropractors and even bone setters. When the treatment is administered by doctors or consultants, it is termed 'surgical' manipulation — a slightly misleading description because, of course, no surgery, in its accepted sense, is involved.

Manipulation alone cannot usually provide a permanent cure for a slipped disc, though it sometimes can afford temporary relief if during the process the prolapsed disc loses contact with the nerve root. A sudden movement by the patient however, usually causes the prolapsed disc to revert to its former position where it again strikes the nerve root and the painful symptoms will re-occur.

However, 'surgical' manipulation, as I use it, plays a vital part in my treatment. Once the disc has been detached, the deformity arising as a result of muscle spasm in the affected area pulling the spinal column to one side, must be corrected. As well as scoliosis, increased kyphosis or exaggerated lordosis may be present, or even a subluxation of the facet joints. All these conditions respond favourably to 'surgical' manipulation. I actually start manipulation to correct deformity during the first treatment, thereby taking advantage of the effect of the local anaesthetic injected to relax the muscles. This flaccidity of the muscles lasts over 4–5 minutes. Generally speaking, I am, in each case, gently rotating the spinal column until the spine assumes its normal alignment. Care must be taken not to over-correct the deformity initially, in order that the contracted ligaments and intrinsic muscles are not torn or damaged. As the treatments proceed, the muscles themselves are no longer constantly spastic due, of course, to the absence of the pressure of the disc on the nerve root. The muscles are also being exercised and toned up by the routine programme prescribed, so that eventually manipulation becomes freer and the deformity is completely corrected.

A more detailed description of the manipulation process, which, of course, varies for each segment of the spinal column (and even at times for each individual), is described in the next Chapters under the appropriate heading.

4. **The Routine Training Programme**

The Fourth part of my treatment is the prescription of a routine programme of exercises. These again vary for each condition and for each individual, because sometimes a combination of the exercises is necessary if the condition is longstanding. These are described in detail in the following Chapters, the relevant programme prescribed for each condition.

The exercises are designed specifically to set in action those muscles which have been in spasm because of the pressure of the disc on the nerve root. Muscles that are in spasm are not in tone. Thus they must be exercised to strengthen them, in order to make the muscles on each side of the spinal column equal in strength, and together strong enough to support the back and head in their normal alignment. Initially, the vertebral bodies of the spinal column articulating with one another are responsible for the contour and shape of the spinal column; but the maintenance of this shape is due entirely to the tone of the muscles which support the column.

Special exercises in the training programme have been devised to take the place of traction — the very common current practice of treating a slipped disc in hospitals. I call this **'Muscle Toning Traction'.** These exercises have the advantage that they can be carried out at home by the patient, thus releasing hospital staff and amenities. They can, therefore, be practised much more frequently and for greater lengths of time, depending on the motivation and the condition of the patient. These exercises are designed specifically to produce a slight extension of the spinal column through the waist line, as well as bringing muscles, previously in spasm, back into action.

Other exercises in the training programme have been devised to produce a rotation of the spinal column. Not only do these tone up the muscles of the column, but also have the effect of compressing it, thus extruding further portions of disc through the tear in the annular ligament.

Following the non-surgical detachment of the disc and the necessary manipulation, the appropriate training programme is demonstrated to the patient so that the exercises can be carried out at regular intervals prior to the next consultation. The full range of exercises is described in detail in the chapter that describes the particular disc lesion being treated (see Chapters V, VI, VII and Appendix II).

After the treatment, I usually give the patient two paracetamol tablets which serve to dull any pain without involving the higher centres of the brain. He (or she) is recommended to take a paracetamol tablet every four hours during the day, with two at night if the pain returns. The patient is also warned that, although he may feel alright on the day of the treatment, the following day he may feel as though he had played a strenuous game of sport at the beginning of the season. He will feel sore, for muscles have been brought into action which have been inactive for a considerable time. However, this is a simple physiological pain which will gradually disappear.

As a rule, treatment is given over a period of two weeks, consisting of three, or at the most four, visits. This is the situation in 92% of cases. Of the remaining 8%, treatment will be required for a few weeks more and of these, 2% may take a month or two to clear up completely. These latter cases are usually ones which have remained untreated for a considerable time and also patients over fifty years old often take longer for their symptoms to disappear. In most cases, these residual symptoms are caused by, firstly, resistant scoliosis, (or torticollis), that will eventually respond to further 'surgical' manipulation and constant practice of the training programme; and/or secondly, by the recurring vibrations of the nerve root made hypersensitive by the mechanical pressure of the prolapsed disc. This latter is like a blow on the chin, which remains sensitive long after a blow has passed. Once the cause of all these symptoms has been removed by detaching the disc, then the symptoms themselves will disappear in due course. Patients must have patience and must continue with the prescribed training programme that has been set out for them. If they fail to do this, then they are simply delaying their complete recovery.

Crash Course Treatment

If a patient comes from overseas or a distant part of the country, I treat this patient with what I call a **Crash Course.** This involves the patient staying in a nearby hotel and visiting me for treatment twice a day. The treatment is carried out over three days on average. The patient then returns home. In some cases, he returns for one day for a final check up a month later, but usually this is unnecessary. Only the very acute cases, for example a patient who is immobile because of acute pain, is advised to stay in a Nursing Home.

Throughout the crash course treatment, a close watch is kept on the patient's physical state and each patient is usually encouraged to perform his particular set of exercises every hour. A high rate of success is achieved with this kind of patient also.

Accidental Cure

One last point I should like to mention here, is the spontaneous cure of a patient who has a spinal disc lesion. Such cures are rare, but they do happen. Some patients may have a very acute disc lesion with all its secondary symptoms, and they are thus practically unable to move. However, such patients, on occasion, do have to rise from bed or from a chair. If they should trip or fall, this usually gives rise to agonising pain in the affected area. When they eventually get up, they may find their pain gone or greatly diminished. What has happened here is that the disc, which had prolapsed and was striking a nerve root, because of the sudden jerk or fall, has been cut off by the sharp edges of the torn annular ligament. It has become detached from its nutrient supply and has fallen away from the nerve root. The disc will atrophy and no longer cause pain, but the deformity resulting from the disc lesion in most cases persists. This kind of cure, however dramatic in effect, is somewhat drastic and cannot honestly be recommended to anyone!

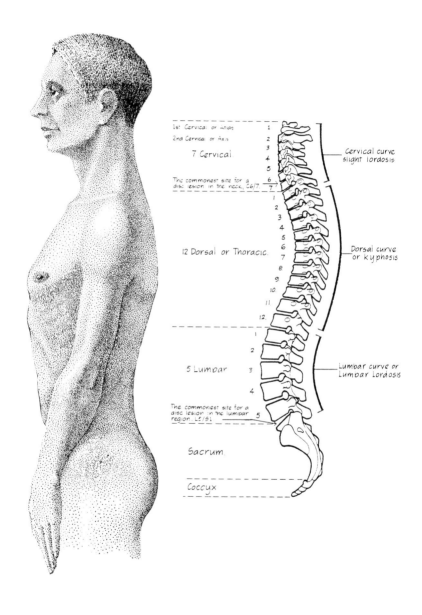

1st Cervical or Atlas   1
2nd Cervical or Axis   2

7 Cervical   3 4 5

Cervical curve
slight lordosis

The commonest site for a
disc lesion in the neck, C6/7.   6 7

12 Dorsal or Thoracic.   1 2 3 4 5 6 7 8 9 10. 11. 12.

Dorsal curve
or kyphosis

5 Lumbar   1 2 3 4

Lumbar curve or
Lumbar lordosis

The commonest site for a
disc lesion in the lumbar
region, L5/S1   5

Sacrum.

Coccyx

Diag. 33. Lateral view of the normal spine.

80

CHAPTER V

Diagnosis and Treatment of a Slipped Disc Lesion in the Lumbar Region

1. My Method of Diagnosis as applied to Patients with Lumbar Pain

Patient's History The routine details of the patient's name, address etc. are taken and, working from the description of this present attack to the descriptions of previous ones, I note the whole history of the condition.

The Neurological Examination will confirm the presence or absence of the ankle reflex. Should the ultimate diagnosis point to a disc lesion condition, the absence of the ankle reflex will indicate a disc lesion at the level L.5/S.1, whereas its presence will indicate the lesion is at a higher level.

Inspection does not, as a rule, yield much information that is helpful in making a differential diagnosis of low back pain. The patient's posture should always be considered, since a faulty posture predisposes to strain and may often result in deformity especially in the lumbar region. The presence of muscle spasm and of lateral and/or anteroposterior deviation of the spinal column, gives some information as to the acuteness of the condition and possible position of a disc lesion, but does not provide enough evidence for a firm diagnosis.

Palpation undertaken systematically, working towards the most sensitive area pointed out by the patient, reveals the position of muscle spasm. This localised tenderness, as elsewhere in the body, usually means a lesion is present in that particular area.

81

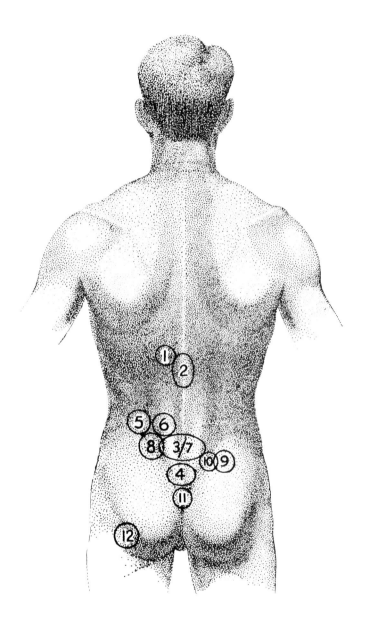

Diag. 34. Differential diagnosis of pain in the lumbar region.

X-rays must be arranged if considered absolutely necessary for diagnosis.

Thus the consultant will now have assessed the severity of the condition and the exact position of greatest pain, but positive diagnosis cannot be made until all the conditions with similar or overlapping symptoms have been considered. This is the differential diagnosis, mentioned earlier.

Differential Diagnosis of Pain in the Lumbar Region

The paragraph numbers which follow relate to the numbers in the diagram opposite.

1. Tenderness over the costovertebral angle may indicate the presence of some genito-urinary lesion, as well as an injury to the transverse process of the first lumbar vertebra. A slipped disc lesion may be present between D.12/L.1.

2. Tenderness of the posterior spinous process and interspinous ligaments, together with a deviation of the posterior spinous process may indicate a fracture which may include the vertebral bodies or disease of these structures. X-ray is essential to eliminate a possible fracture or bone disease. Tenderness of the interspinous ligaments is indicative of acute strain or sprain due to faulty posture. A slipped disc lesion may be present between D.12/L.1 or more rarely between L.1/L.2.

3. Tenderness in the region of the articular facets between L.5/S.1 may be due to lumbosacral sprain from a hyperflexion or hyperextension injury. It may be due to a muscle sprain since the erectores spinae overlie the facets here. However, this type of injury is usually accompanied by a disc lesion.

4. Pain and tenderness in the dorsum of the sacrum commonly produces exaggerated lumbo-sacral lordosis.

5. Tenderness in the region of the iliac crest may indicate a slipped disc lesion between L.1/L.2 but may also be due to the sprain of the origin of the iliocostalis muscle.

6. Tenderness or pain at the point of the ilio-lumbar angle may be due to the fracture of the transverse process at this level; a strain of the ilio-lumbar ligaments due to faulty posture; or acute sprain of the erector spinae or a disc lesion at L.4/L.5.

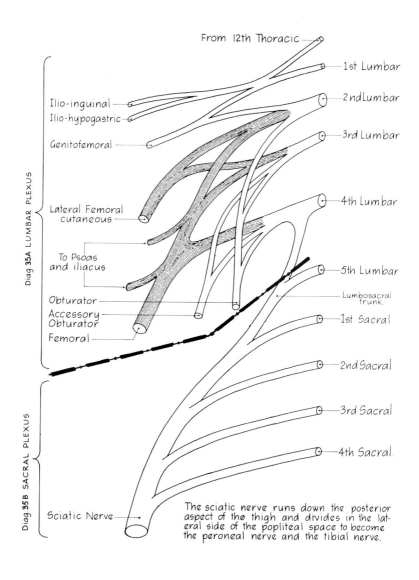

From 12th Thoracic

1st Lumbar

Ilio-inguinal
Ilio-hypogastric

2nd Lumbar

Genitofemoral

3rd Lumbar

Diag 35A LUMBAR PLEXUS

Lateral Femoral
cutaneous

4th Lumbar

To Psoas
and iliacus

5th Lumbar

Lumbosacral
trunk.

Obturator
Accessory
Obturator
Femoral

1st Sacral

2nd Sacral

Diag 35B SACRAL PLEXUS

3rd Sacral

4th Sacral.

Sciatic Nerve

The sciatic nerve runs down the posterior
aspect of the thigh and divides in the lateral side of the popliteal space to become
the peroneal nerve and the tibial nerve.

Diag. 35. Showing the plan of lumbar and sacral plexus.

84

7. Tenderness of the spinous processes of the 5th lumbar and 1st sacral vertebra is usually caused by faulty posture and frequently in spina bifida occulta with the ununited spinous process of the 1st sacral vertebra. It may also indicate a disc lesion at L.5/S.1.

8. Sensitivity in the area of the posterior iliac crest and posterior superior iliac spine may indicate muscle strain or sprain or a disc lesion at L.5/S.1.

9. Tenderness at the sacro-sciatic notch usually indicates a lesion in the sacro-iliac region. This is fairly common in football or rugby injuries.

10. Sensitivity in the area of the sacro-iliac joint, i.e. the region between the posterior superior spine and the posterior inferior spine, is usually due to sacro-iliac strain or sprain.

11. Tenderness of the ligaments at the sacro-coccygeal junction is usually due to sacro-coccygeal injury, either a strain, sprain or a fracture.

12. Tenderness showing involvement of the sciatic nerve, midway between the greater trochanter and ischial tuberosity at the level of the gluteal fold, indicates hypersensitivity of the sciatic nerve trunk which may accompany either a lumbar or sacro-iliac condition, the commonest of which is a slipped disc lesion between L.5/S.1 vertebral bodies.

All these symptoms and the conditions associated with them have to be considered before the examiner is certain of his diagnosis. However, if he considers a disc lesion in the lumbar region is present, it is then necessary to establish the exact position of the lesion.

Diagnosis and Treatment of a Slipped Disc Lesion in the Lumbar Region

The commonest sites of a slipped disc lesion in the whole of the spinal column are in the lumbar area, the most common being in the lowest lumbar area, i.e. between L.5 and S.1. The symptoms vary according to the site of the lesion. From a clinical point of view a slipped disc condition in the lumbar area may be divided into four specific areas:

1. Disc lesion between L.5/S.1
2. Disc lesion between L.4/5
3. Disc lesion between L.2/3, L.3/4
4. Disc lesion between L.1/2

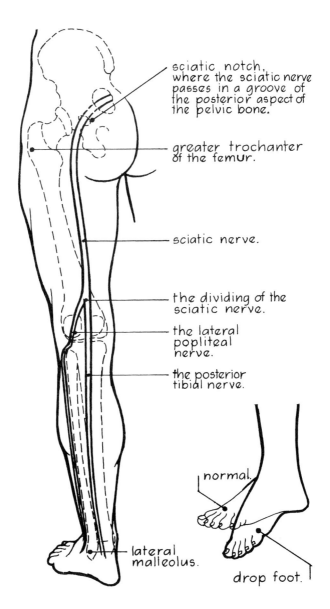

sciatic notch, where the sciatic nerve passes in a groove of the posterior aspect of the pelvic bone.

greater trochanter of the femur.

sciatic nerve.

the dividing of the sciatic nerve.

the lateral popliteal nerve.

the posterior tibial nerve.

normal.

drop foot.

lateral malleolus.

Diag. 36. Showing the whole length of the sciatic nerve, the longest nerve in the body.

Symptoms of a Disc Lesion between L.5/S.1

This is the commonest site for a disc lesion in the spinal column due to the sharp angulation between the fifth lumbar vertebra and the superior aspect of the sacrum. In the erect posture the whole weight of the trunk bears down on this angulation, causing a tremendous strain on the annular ligament which holds the disc in position. The weakest point of the annular ligament is at its postero-lateral aspect where it is thinnest and unprotected by the posterior longitudinal ligament and it is at this site that the disc most commonly prolapses. This area is closest to the spinal nerve roots. Thus the prolapsed disc in this position will, as a rule, strike the **sciatic nerve.** Pain will radiate on the affected site from the lowest area of the back, through the centre of the buttock and then pass down the posterior aspect of the thigh towards the lateral aspect of the popliteal space. At this point the sciatic nerve divides; one branch called the posterior tibial nerve passes straight down the centre of the calf to the lateral malleolus; the other branch known as the lateral popliteal nerve winds round the neck of the fibula and runs downwards over the dorsum of the foot and toes. Pain may occur along the lines of all these nerve tracts or may be felt simply in the lower lumbar region, into the buttock, missing the thigh altogether but striking down the lateral aspect of the leg to the foot. Sometimes the pressure of the disc on the sciatic nerve results in temporary paralysis or **'drop foot'** (see diagram opposite). Other symptoms may reveal themselves once the more acute pain has cleared up and may not appear to be present until a two-week period has elapsed. The commonest are burning sensations which may be followed by pins and needles, especially in the toes and usually, once these symptoms have cleared up, a patchy numbness may be discovered in the same area. This latter symptom, numbness, in the minority of cases in which it occurs, may last for some months, but will eventually clear up completely and, as a rule, never returns.

The ankle reflex is usually absent. Indication of its presence again usually means that the disc has cleared off the nerve root.

A slight degree of scoliosis is present in 50% of cases, due to muscle spasm extending upwards from the gluteal area. The muscles, which are in spasm on the affected side will, in turn, pull the pelvis upwards, giving rise to a slight to moderate tilting of the pelvis with the same degree of scoliosis. The pelvis on the affected side will, in turn, bring the lower limb up with it, thus causing an apparent shortening of that limb, but if the limbs are measured lengthwise from

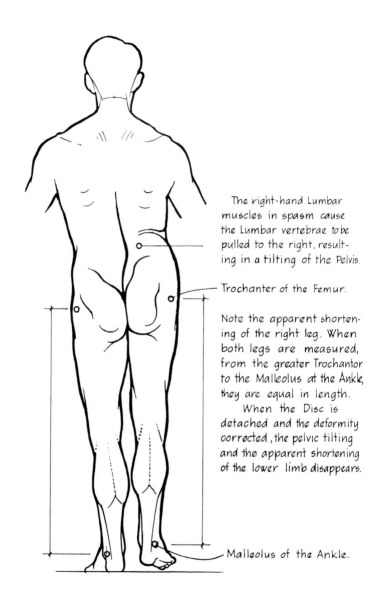

The right-hand Lumbar muscles in spasm cause the Lumbar vertebrae to be pulled to the right, resulting in a tilting of the Pelvis.

Trochanter of the Femur.

Note the apparent shortening of the right leg. When both legs are measured, from the greater Trochantor to the Malleolus at the Ankle, they are equal in length.

When the Disc is detached and the deformity corrected, the pelvic tilting and the apparent shortening of the lower limb disappears.

Malleolus of the Ankle.

Diag. 37. Posterior view of the back showing scoliosis to the right as a result of slipped disc lesion in the lumbar area.

the greater trochanter of the femur to the lateral malleolus of the ankle joint on either side, they will be of similar length. When the condition, which initially produced the spasm and tilting of the pelvis is cleared up, the lower limb will look similar in length to the unaffected side and the pelvis become horizontal. It is interesting to note that out of 2,000 cases, with no back trouble whatsoever, only 10-15% of lower limbs were found to be absolutely equal in length in the same individual.

Symptoms of a Disc Lesion Between L.4/5

The next most common site for a disc lesion is between L.4 and L.5. This is due to the moderate angulation between these two vertebral bodies, particularly in females, and, as in lumbar L.5/S.1 disc lesions, the downward pressure of the trunk has a specific bearing on the occurrence of disc lesions at this site. The disc usually prolapses at the postero-lateral aspect of the annular ligament where it is weakest and also nearest to the spinal nerve roots. The nerve commonly struck at this level is the fourth lumbar nerve which is the largest member of the lumbar plexus of nerves. This causes all muscles supplied by it to go into a very acute spasm, giving rise to very severe pain in the mid-lumbar region, and may extend into the gluteal region to a lesser degree. These muscles in extreme spasm will pull the spinal column towards them, giving rise to a severe lumbar scoliosis. If the erector spinati, the powerful muscles on either side of the spinal column, are also affected they will go into spasm and pull the spinal column backwards, giving rise to a flattening of the lumbar lordosis and, at times, a complete reversal i.e. a lumbar kyphosis. There is often an overlapping of these deformities and the patient may suffer from a gross distortion of the spinal column.

From a clinical point of view, the presence or absence of the ankle jerks is a most important indicator of the exact site of the disc lesion. The ankle reflex, as a rule is always present in lumber 4/5 lesions but absent if the lesion is between L.5/S.1.

In a minority of cases, acute pain is experienced from the groin to just above the knee joint on the affected side. This is due to mechanical pressure of the disc on the femoral nerve, producing a **Femoral Neuritis.**

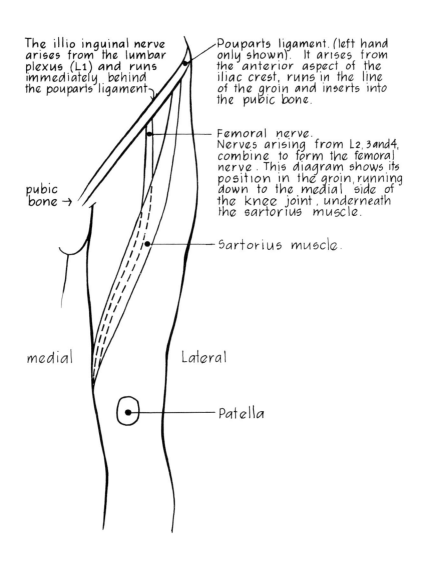

The illio inguinal nerve arises from the lumbar plexus (L1) and runs immediately behind the pouparts ligament

Pouparts ligament. (left hand only shown). It arises from the anterior aspect of the iliac crest, runs in the line of the groin and inserts into the pubic bone.

Femoral nerve.
Nerves arising from L2,3and4, combine to form the femoral nerve. This diagram shows its position in the groin, running down to the medial side of the knee joint, underneath the sartorius muscle.

pubic bone →

Sartorius muscle.

medial

Lateral

Patella

Diag. 38. Section of upper leg showing position of femoral nerve and ilio-inguinal nerve.

90

The Symptoms of a Disc Lesion between L.2/3 and L.3/4

Disc lesions at these sites are not common but do occur, particularly as a result of motor car accidents involving a whiplash injury. The disc, prolapsing through the postero-lateral aspect of the annular ligament may strike the nerve root between L.2/3 and L.3/4. Acute pain will be experienced in the mid lumbar region with a slight to moderate scoliosis to the affected side, with at times, a flattening of the normal lumbar lordosis and, in extreme cases, a kyphosis in this region. Hypersensitivity may be felt from the groin down the anterior aspect of the thigh to the knee joint level. This is due to femoral nerve involvement, giving rise to a **Femoral Neuritis.**

The Symptoms of a Slipped Disc Lesion Between L.1/2

This is an uncommon site for a disc lesion, and, as a rule, it is due to direct trauma, such as a motor car accident or a rugby football accident. If the disc, prolapsing through the thin postero-lateral aspect of the annular ligament, strikes the first lumbar nerve, which forms part of the lumbar plexus then **Ilio-Inguinal Neuritis** will occur. Pain will radiate from the upper lumbar region, around the brim of the pelvis, along the inguinal canal area to the region of the pelvic bone on the affected side.

Quite often this condition is incorrectly diagnosed as an inguinal or femoral hernia.

The Non-Surgical Detachment of Disc in the Lumbar Region

I always examine my patients in the erect posture with their back towards me and clothing removed from the affected site. I always avoid the straight leg-raising test which is commonly carried out by most of my colleagues because, in sciatic cases, in particular, the stretching of this already hypersensitive nerve only acutely aggravates the condition. See diagram 39.

A very careful study of the normal spinal contour and a detailed assessment of the patient's symptoms should enable any abnormality to be detected. The spinal column will usually be twisted or pulled over to one side and, by palpating the affected area, the muscles will be felt to be quite hard or in real spasm. When a lesion occurs in the lower lumbar area, the erector spinatus, the long, powerful muscle

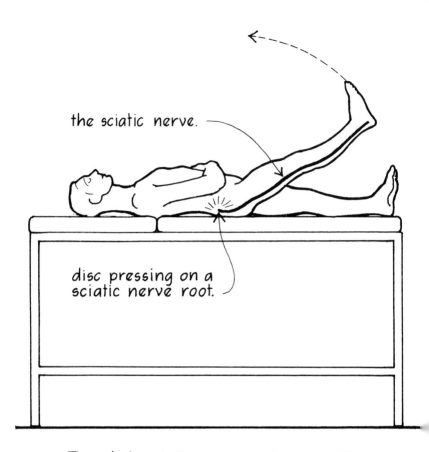

the sciatic nerve.

disc pressing on a
sciatic nerve root.

The whole sciatic nerve is hypersensitive.
Thus by carrying out the straight leg
raising test one is stretching the nerve
thereby increasing the sciatica.

This test should be avoided.

Diag. 39. Straight leg raising test.

lying on either side of the spinal column, is usually affected, with involvement of the underlying muscle groups and this spasm may extend into the gluteal area, i.e. the buttock itself.

I now examine the patient to identify the exact nerve root which is involved. Using a heavy pointed rubber tendon reflex hammer I tap along the line of the erector spinatus. When the area is tapped at the exact site of the disc lesion a slight flickering of muscle occurs, causing the patient literally to jump with the severity of the pain. I usually continue with the hammer right down the sacrum and then return back upwards to check again for the area of greatest spasticity. Having decided on the exact site, I make a small ring in red pencil over the area.

The presence of scoliosis is usually apparent but is also tested by flexing the patient laterally towards the affected side. This may cause great pain because when I do this, I am simply aggravating the condition. On the other hand, when I flex the patient away from the spastic area — that is, laterally in the opposite direction — there will be movement with very little pain. The reason for the acute pain on lateral flexion of the spinal column to the affected side is due to the compressing of the vertebral bodies towards one another, which causes increased bulging of the annular ligament. In these circumstances, more of the disc is usually pushed through the tear in the annular ligament, increasing the pressure on the nerve root and causing an increase of pain. On the other hand lateral flexion in the reverse direction causes the disc to be pulled laterally away from the tear, causing diminished pressure on the sensitive nerve root.

I then physically press through the muscle group which is in spasm with my thumb, usually causing some degree of discomfort to the patient. If, for example, I am dealing with the left side of the patient, I put my right hand on his or her right shoulder and flex the spinal column laterally, pulling it with my right hand towards the right. This opens up the space between the lateral processes at the site of the disc lesion. This permits me with my left thumb to press very firmly over the site of the disc and brings my thumb on to the disc itself. Continuing to press forward with my left thumb, I keep pulling the patient down laterally with my right hand on his or her shoulder. This lateral flexion of the column separates the lateral processes of the spinal vertebrae and gives me access to the disc complex area. The patient is left in this position, that is, in the erect posture, with the spinal column laterally flexed to the right to a fair degree. A sterile syringe, already charged with a few drops of novocaine or other local anaesthetic, is then inserted through the skin which has been already cleaned with surgical spirit. The needle is guided down between the

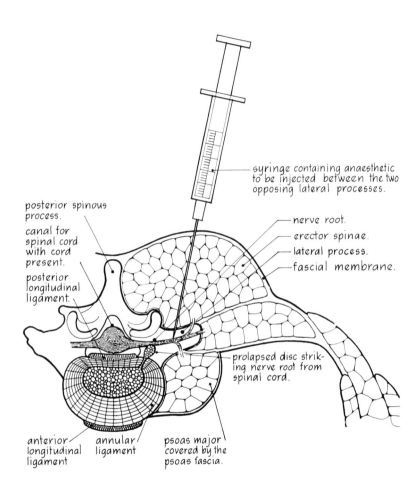

posterior spinous process.

canal for spinal cord with cord present.

posterior longitudinal ligament.

syringe containing anaesthetic to be injected between the two opposing lateral processes.

nerve root.

erector spinae.

lateral process.

fascial membrane.

prolapsed disc striking nerve root from spinal cord.

anterior longitudinal ligament

annular ligament

psoas major covered by the psoas fascia.

Diag. 40. The injection of local anaesthesia into the affected nerve root to achieve 'Nerve Root Block'.

lateral processes — say between L.4/5, if this should be the position of the diagnosed disc lesion. A twitching of the muscles will confirm when the needle has touched the optimum location for the injection. I then inject straight into the compressed nerve root (or into the nerve tract, as close as is practical to its emergence though the intraverted foramen). As a result of this, the muscles which were in spasm become soft and flaccid. I continue to inject slowly into the nerve root, eventually withdrawing the needle. This local anaesthetic will only last 3 to 5 minutes but the muscles that were in spasm become soft and quite flaccid almost immediately. This allows me, by firm pressure with my left thumb, to pass through the soft muscle area straight on to the disc. I then locate with my thumb the disc from above and press downwards. I can actually feel that portion of disc, which is protruding between the vertebral bodies, being detached. The torn edge of the annular ligament is quite firm and sharp and so when the disc, being of a soft gelatinous material, is compressed against its lower aspect it is easily detached or broken off.

I do not put my patients to bed following this non-surgical procedure. They are instructed to keep moving about as though nothing had been done. If there is any more disc to come out it will do so during this gentle activity and can be dealt with in exactly the same manner as already described, at the next appointment. Normally it takes two weeks for the condition to clear up from the first detachment of disc. The remainder of the disc, if any, should be left to worm its way out from between the vertebral bodies until all the disc has been cleared away during the course of treatment.

This is a description of the Non-Surgical Technique for the detachment of a lumbar disc lesion. Some deformity may have arisen because of the lesion and this is now treated, both by 'surgical' manipulation and a course of training exercises.

Treatment of the Deformity in the Lumbar Region by Surgical Manipulation

Having cleared away one of the patient's problems, I see no point in leaving him deformed for the rest of his life. The deformity that has arisen because of the slipped spinal disc, must now be treated. There may be scoliosis: there may also be a loss of the normal lumbar lordosis (i.e. the hollow in the lower lumbar region); or instead of their being the normal lumbar curve or flattening of the curve, the

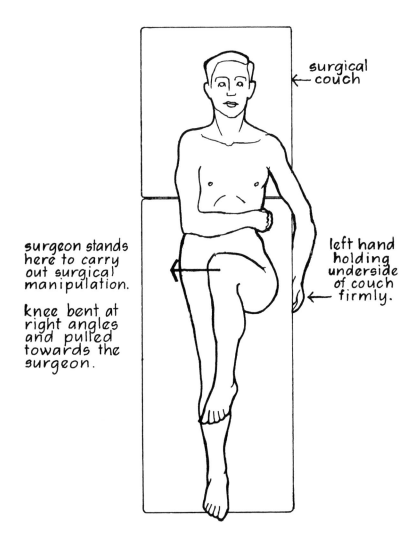

surgical
couch

surgeon stands
here to carry
out surgical
manipulation.

knee bent at
right angles
and pulled
towards the
surgeon.

left hand
holding
underside
of couch
firmly.

Diag. 41. Surgical manipulation to correct deformity, i.e. scoliosis, in the
lumbar region.

curve may actually be reversed so that the lumbar area of the spinal column protrudes backwards instead of going into the normal hollow.

The treatment is similar in most cases but, of course, it depends to some extent on how long the deformity has been present. If it has been present for only two or three weeks it may require no treatment at all, but where a patient has been deformed for a lengthy period, 'surgical' manipulation is very important and undertaken whilst the local anaesthetic is still effective. The patient lies on the orthopaedic couch flat on his back. If he has a scoliosis curve to the right, then with the right side of his body to me I raise the left leg with the knee bent and bring it over towards me. The patient is told to hold onto the under edge of the couch with his left hand. Then I gently rotate the pelvis towards me and thus the curve of the spinal column which came towards me is now being pulled away from me. In other words I start straightening up the patient's spinal column. Audible clicking may occur. This is caused by one bony facet clicking over another and, occasionally, to the breaking down of adhesions which may have formed if the patient has been deformed for a considerable time. This clicking sound is not due, as I have explained, to the replacing of a disc, for because of its gelatinous nature, such a sound could not be produced. Similarly, patients are often told by the manipulator that he is putting the disc back into place. This again is not possible because the disc would disintegrate if pressure were exerted on it in order to replace it. Even if such a technique were devised, there would be no means of preventing the disc prolapsing once more through the annular ligament. In reality, one good cough or sneeze would provide sufficient pressure to cause the disc to prolapse once again.

During my treatment I only correct the spinal alignment to a minimum degree at the first visit. I make no attempt to complete the correction in chronic cases. If one does so, one may tear the contracted intrinsic ligaments and muscles and aggravate the whole condition. One session of manipulation is usually completed within ten seconds.

In cases where the sciatic nerve is also involved, the patient remains lying, still on his back on the couch. I then bend the affected leg at the knee and with very, very firm pressure I press my thumbs straight into the sciatic nerve itself, pressing firmly on the nerve at intervals of about every two inches right down the whole tract of the nerve to the foot. By doing this, one will in most cases stop the vibrations which continue even though the disc has been detached. When a nerve is struck, like a punch on the jaw, the blow may have passed but the area struck may remain hypersensitive for a few weeks.

Another example will make this clearer. When a note is struck on a piano, the string will go on vibrating for some considerable time after the fingers are removed. To stop these vibrations of the piano string, one mechanically presses down the damper pedal. This is exactly what is being done when I physically press on the sciatic nerve. Similarly, if femoral neuritis is present, I press down firmly with my thumbs along the whole length of the vibrating femoral nerve. If ilio-inguinal neuritis is present, nerve pain will extend along the iliac crest, into the inguinal canal and then to the pubic bone, and this is similarly treated.

Some further discomfort will be felt on the day following treatment — muscular pains similar to those experienced after the first day of sport in the new season. This pain is purely physiological and will soon pass away now that muscles which have lain inactive, are now being exercised. I prescribe two paracetamols to be taken, every four hours if necessary.

As already mentioned, most of my patients are as good as new within two weeks and this statement is correct in over 90% of true slipped spinal disc cases, without gross deformity. A small percentage of cases, depending on how long the problem has been there, will continue to have a degree of slight scoliosis and sciatica if the sciatic nerve has been involved. The sciatic pain usually clears up quite quickly but the patient may be left with a tingling, or pins and needles sensation, or there may be a numbness present in the affected limb, especially in the region of the foot. This numbness is usually the last symptom to disappear and it may take several weeks or months to clear up completely. However, during this period the patient's mobility is unimpaired.

The Training Programme for Lumbar Disc Lesions

Muscles that are in spasm caused by the mechanical pressure of the disc on the nerve root supplying those muscles, are not in good tone. Thus I prescribe a training programme to regain tone in the affected muscles. The prescribed exercises must not be neglected, for the muscles must eventually be toned up to support the back in its correct alignment. The daily performance of the exercises contained in this programme calls for some patience and perseverance if the condition is longstanding. It must always be remembered that muscles will quickly lose their tone if they are not kept active and that oxygen is essential for muscle building, so deep breaths must be taken when performing the exercises.

EXERCISE I: **Muscle Toning Traction**

For patients with lumbar disc lesions I advocate what I describe as 'Muscle Toning Traction'. This exercise was developed by me as a far better way of producing traction on muscles than the conventional and varied forms of traction carried out as a matter of routine in our hospitals today. This exercise has the advantage that it can be carried out at home by the patient, thus releasing hospital staff and amenities. It can also be practised much more frequently and for greater lengths of time depending on the motivation and condition of the patient.

The exercise involves folding the arms in front of the chest, raising the shoulders to the ears and, with head held backwards and eyes to the ceiling, moving the chest laterally. This will move the spinal column from side to side for about two inches in either direction. In effect, the patient will gradually pull himself up and up all the time, thus producing a slight extension of the spinal column through the waist line. This has the further effect of bringing muscles previously inactive back into action. In other words the patient is toning muscles that were in spasm but not in tone, and getting the two sides balanced. Patients are instructed to perform this movement fifty times, moving like a pendulum no more than two inches on either side.

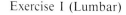

Exercise I (Lumbar)

Muscle Toning Traction

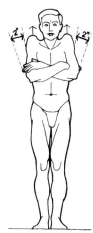

1. Stand erect with feet together.
2. Expand chest — this increases lumbar curve.
3. Fold arms across chest.
4. Raise points of shoulders to ears.
5. In this posture move the chest for 2″ from side to side 25 times each way, bending through waist.
6. Take a deep breath with each movement. The shoulders should remain fixed in this position. It is the chest which moves from side to side and at the same time it is being pulled upwards all the time.

Diag. 42

99

EXERCISE II: **Spinal Rotation**

As well as Muscle Toning Traction, I usually advocate Spinal Rotation through the lumbar region. The patient should adopt the same position as in the previous exercise. He then rotates the chest through the waistline round and round no more than 2″ from vertical — first twenty times in one direction and then twenty times in the other direction. This method of extension and movement of the muscles should be done four times a day and, in severe cases, every hour.

Rotation Exercises of this nature form an important part of my non-surgical technique. When the body is rotated, the spinal column on the affected side, is alternately extended and compressed, thus allowing the residual pieces of disc to pass through the tear in the annular ligament, the sharp edges of which cut off the pieces of disc.

Naturally, these rotation exercises are also designed to tone up the muscles and ligaments which relate to rotary movement.

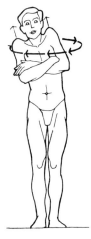

Exercise II (Lumbar)

Spinal Rotation

1. Adopt the same posture as in Exercise I.
2. Rotate the chest through the waistline round and round for no more than 2″ from the vertical — first 20 times in one direction and then 20 times in the other direction.

Diag. 43.

EXERCISE III: **Pendulum Movement of Trunk**

The patient should stand in the erect posture with the arms kept at the sides of the body, and expand the chest which increases the lumbar lordosis. In this posture, he should flex the trunk laterally for two inches to either side at speed, counting fifty i.e. 25 to either side. This should take no more than one minute and should be carried out four times a day.

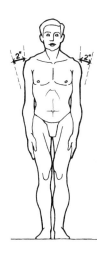

Exercise III (Lumbar)

Pendulum Movement of the Trunk

1. Stand in the erect posture with the arms kept at the side of the body.
2. Keep the chest expanded, which increases the lumbar lordosis.
3. Flex the chest laterally 25 times from side to side, 2″ in either direction at speed. Bend at waist only. Do not move legs. The shoulders are held fixed and only move with the chest.

Diag. 44.

EXERCISE IV: Rotation of Trunk through the Waistline

After a few days this exercise also should be carried out four times daily. The patient should rotate the trunk through the waistline, 25 movements in both directions, again bending not more than two inches in from the vertical. In this exercise the arms are kept close to the body; the shoulders should not be raised, but allowed to move with the chest.

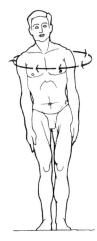

Exercise IV (Lumbar)

Rotation of the Trunk through the Waist Line

1. Stand in the erect posture as in exercise III.
2. Rotate the chest, bending at waist line only, not more than 2″, 25 times in one direction and 25 times in the other.
3. Arms kept close to body.
4. Shoulders are not raised, but move with the chest.

Diag. 45.

101

EXERCISE V: (Lumbar)

If scoliosis is present, this exercise helps to pull the affected muscles out of spasm and straightens the spinal column. In the erect posture, the patient should jerk the pelvis from the affected side straight across to the unaffected side.

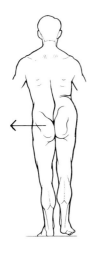

Exercise V

Pelvic Jerk

Jerk the pelvis from the affected side straight across to the unaffected side, i.e. from right to left (for a right sided scoliosis), 20 jerks 4 times per day.

Diag. 46.

As the training programme proceeds, the patient will gradually regain the normal lordosis curve in the lumbar region and the scoliosis will disappear. In over 90% of cases this is achieved within a fortnight. In 2-3% of cases pain may persist or recur over many months.

During the course of treatments, whilst I recommend the patient be mobile, it is also important not to aggravate his condition and thus retard recovery. I have prepared summaries about the various conditions and included them in Appendix II to enable the patient to understand his own condition, to follow the prescribed exercises precisely, and also to understand which activities are to be avoided and those which will help to make him more comfortable. I usually summarise the relevant points in the consulting room before he leaves.

Apart from the exercises, patients are instructed to take things easily until a fortnight has elapsed. However, they must keep gently active throughout the day, resisting the temptation to lie down until bedtime. With regard to sleeping, many practitioners recommend an orthopaedic bed or a piece of hardboard inserted under the mattress, but I deplore such advice. A good interior sprung mattress provides

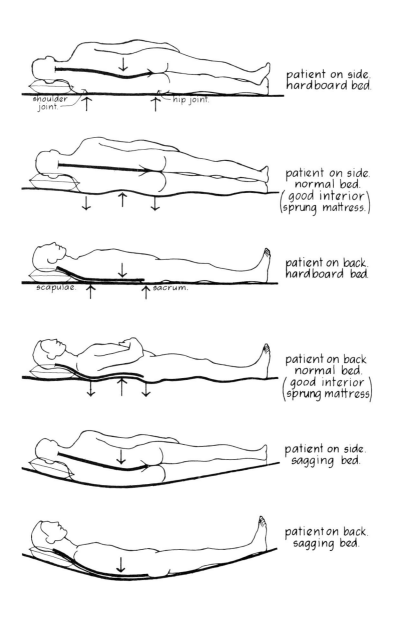

patient on side.
hardboard bed.

shoulder joint.   hip joint.

patient on side.
normal bed.
(good interior)
(sprung mattress.)

patient on back.
hardboard bed.

scapulae.   sacrum.

patient on back
normal bed.
(good interior)
(sprung mattress)

patient on side.
sagging bed.

patient on back.
sagging bed.

Diag. 47. Sleeping postures.

103

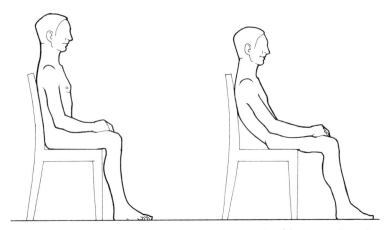

The correct way to sit on a chair. The lumbar curve is well supported.

Patients should never sit on the front edge of a chair as this causes the lumbar curve to be reversed.

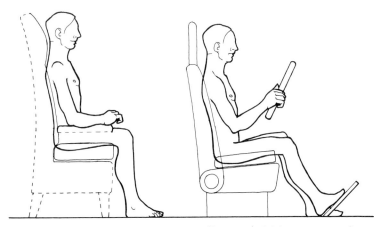

An easy chair should be upright with a well sprung back and seat. The patient should sit with his buttocks well back into the seat, (use additional cushions if necessary) and with his feet flat on the floor. The thighs should be at right-angles to the leg, with no pressure from the seat behind the knee joint.

The ideal driving posture for a back sufferer. Ensure the buttocks are well back, the driving wheel is close to the body, and the legs are always slightly flexed. Use a good, thick, well upholstered, latex-foam cushion on seat, and at the back. Use additional cushions, if necessary.

Diag. 48. Seating postures to alleviate lower lumbar pain.

cushioning for the taut muscles in spasm and enables the bony prominences of the spinal column (for example the point of the shoulder and the protruding hip bone) to be impaled into the mattress, thus allowing the spinal column to retain its normal contour during sleep, and to be supported throughout its full length.

Similarly, a patient should avoid sitting on a hard seat, especially if sciatica is present, for his condition is aggravated by the weight of the trunk pressing down on the sensitive nerve and pressing it against the bony sciatic notch of the pelvis. The use of a small feather or latex foam cushion will prevent this. A patient should, for the same reason, avoid sitting with his buttock on the edge of the chair. He should sit straight into the back of the chair, to avoid bending his back so much that normal lordosis is reversed. Most modern easy chairs do not conform in depth to the average length of the human thigh and thus do not provide proper support for even a normal healthy person's back. They are also usually too low to allow a patient to rise easily from them. A relatively higher and more upright type of chair with relatively less depth of seat will usually provide both more support and comfort, but this obviously varies according to the size and build of the patient. It is also advisable for the patient to avoid crossing the legs when sitting down, for crossed legs pull on the already sensitive nerve roots.

Drivers of motor cars will also find a small latex foam cushion is beneficial and should try to position their seats so that they avoid stretching unnecessarily to reach the foot pedals (see diagram).

Patients should avoid all types of sport that involve quick jerky movements for at least a fortnight, or until the condition has cleared up. Diving especially may aggravate the condition as it may hyperextend the spinal column. Swimming, however, is a good exercise.

Patients who are keen walkers often ask if walking is a good exercise. I advise them against it. Keen walkers usually take big strides and these aggravate the condition. In acute lumbar disc lesions, which produce spasm of the lower lumbar muscles and possible associated sciatica, each step tends to stretch the lumbar nerve roots or the sciatic nerve itself and, of course, the muscles which are in spasm will also be stretched. Strenuous walking during treatment is therefore not a good exercise. It is best to walk taking very short steps, whether the back is painful or not, until the end of the treatment, when thereafter patients may walk as much as they like.

Patients should avoid standing for any length of time because the weight of the trunk presses down on the hypersensitive nerve root. Relief can be obtained by standing with the body weight on to the

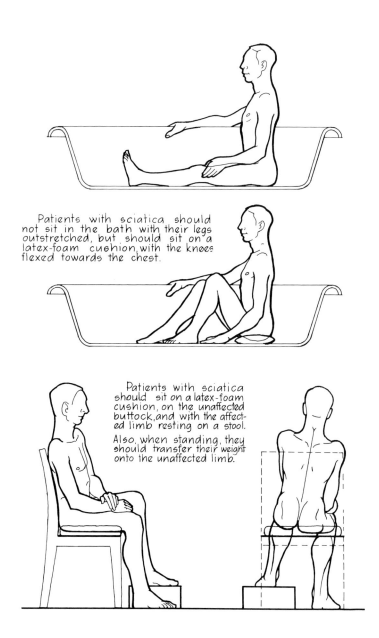

Patients with sciatica should
not sit in the bath with their legs
outstretched, but should sit on a
latex-foam cushion, with the knees
flexed towards the chest.

Patients with sciatica
should sit on a latex-foam
cushion, on the unaffected
buttock, and with the affected limb resting on a stool.

Also, when standing, they
should transfer their weight
onto the unaffected limb.

Diag. 49. Postures recommended to alleviate sciatica.

106

unaffected side and slightly flexing the body laterally to this side.

A patient suffering from sciatica should also try to avoid sitting in a bath where the legs are stretched out at right angles to the body. This is virtually akin to the straight leg-raising test during which the sensitive nerve roots are being stretched. The patient should sit on a small rubber cushion in the bath.

Carrying heavy loads should be avoided especially during the first two weeks of treatment. Patients lifting anything, even the smallest item, should bend the knees, keeping the back straight, and take the full weight in their arms. Patients, when tying shoe laces or putting on socks or tights should sit and draw the feet up towards them rather than bend the back and reach down to floor level. Bending the back forwards to touch the floor should be avoided.

Ladies should not use a vacuum cleaner for at least two weeks, as the pulling backwards and forwards of the cleaner puts a considerable strain on the lumbar muscles, thus aggravating the condition.

Coughing and sneezing should be avoided whenever possible as this causes a wave of pressure of the cerebro-spinal fluid that surrounds the brain and the whole of the spinal cord. This wave will strike the hypersensitive affected nerve root and cause sharp sudden intense pain.

Surgical corsets and plaster casts must not be used as this leads to 'disuse atrophy' in the lumbar muscles. Most patients, in any case, find the use of these frustrating.

Greatest relaxation is obtained for the sciatic nerve if the patient lies on his abdomen with the hip of the affected side hyperextended and the knee joint fully flexed. A small bolster or pillow should be placed under the knee joint.

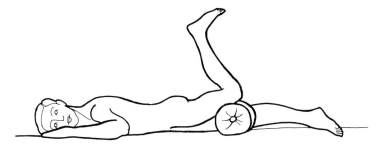

Diag. 50. Relaxation of the sciatic nerve.

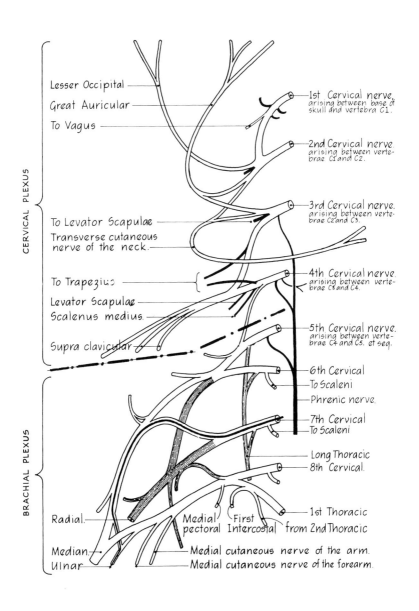

Diag. 51. Nerves of the cervical region.

108

CHAPTER VI

Diagnosis and Treatment of a Slipped Disc Lesion in the Cervical Region

THIS CONDITION is not as common as that in the lumbar area. It is usually caused by an accident which may involve 'whiplash injury', during which the head is suddenly jerked forwards and backwards. This tears the annular ligament at the weakest point, its postero-lateral aspect, and allows the disc to prolapse. The clinical features will depend on precisely where the annular ligament was torn and which nerve in the cervical column has been struck. From a clinical point of view a slipped disc condition in the cervical region should be divided into three specific areas:

1. Disc lesion between C.6/7
2. Disc lesion between C.2/3, 3/4, 4/5 and 5/6
3. Disc lesion between the base of the skull and C.1

However, there may be an overlapping of clinical features in each, which may lead to early confusion in coming to a firm diagnosis. The two most common sites for spinal disc lesions in the neck are between C.6/7 and between the base of the skull and C.1.

1. Symptoms of a Disc Lesion between C.6/7

The prolapsed disc in this position leads to very acute pain at the base of the neck on one side or the other for it is unusual for nerve roots on both sides to be struck at the same time. The muscles supplied by the affected nerve go into spasm which may extend partially up the neck and, at times, downwards affecting the supra-scapular group of muscles and, sometimes also down the medial scapular group of muscles to the lower aspect of the scapula.

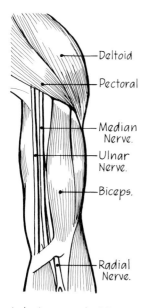

Anterior aspect of the upper arm showing the Ulnar, Median and Radial nerves.

Deltoid

Pectoral

Median Nerve.

Ulnar Nerve.

Biceps.

Radial Nerve.

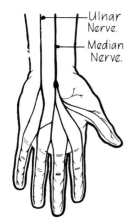

Ulnar Nerve.

Median Nerve.

Lines showing the distribution of Motor and Sensory nerves in the hand.

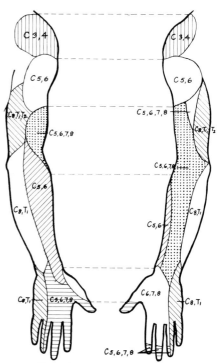

C 3,4

C 5,6

C₈,T₁,T₂

C 5,6,7,8

C 5,6

C₈,T₁

C₈,T₁

C 5,6,7,8

C₈,T₁,T₂

C 5,6,7,8

C 5,6

C₈,T₁

C 6,7,8

C₈,T₁

C 5,6,7,8

The different sensory areas of the arm and hand, the muscles of which are supplied by the nerve-roots indicated.

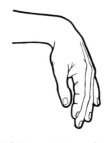

Radial Nerve Palsy, or 'Drop Wrist'

Diag. 52. The ulnar and median nerve, the sensory areas of the arm and hand, and Radial nerve palsy.

110

In most cases the brachial plexus is struck giving rise to brachial neuritis. These nerves supply all the muscle power to the arms. Two larger nerves, the median and ulnar nerves, are most commonly affected. In the case of the ulnar nerve, the pain, following the nerve tract, travels down the inner side of the arm towards the small finger and half of the ring finger. Since the ulnar nerve supplies 15 of the 20 small muscles of the hand, there is, in many cases, marked loss of power in the hand as a whole, with disturbed sensation on the ulnar side of the hand (the hypothenar eminence) and particularly affecting the small finger and the ulnar side of the ring finger.

The other most commonly struck nerve supplying the upper limb, is the median nerve. In this case, pain may be experienced from the base of the neck, down the lateral or radial side of the arm with pain, 'pins or needles' or tingling in the thumb, index, middle finger and half of the ring finger on the thumb side. Weakness may occur in the region of the thumb or thenar eminence, as the median nerve supplies only the remaining five small muscles of the hand, which are in the thumb area. If the whole plexus of the nerve roots is struck there may be 'pins and needles' sensation affecting every finger of the hand as well as loss of muscle power and patchy numbness. The sensory disturbance of the ulnar and median nerves in the hand is not always clearcut.

An infrequent result of a disc lesion affecting the brachial plexus is injury to the radial nerve which gives rise to a 'drop wrist' i.e. **Radial nerve palsy.**

2. Symptoms of a Disc Lesion between Cervical 2/3, 3/4, 4/5 and 5/6

The prolapsed disc in any of these sites striking the nerve roots, particularly of the cervical plexus, leads to acute pain in the affected area with marked spasm of muscles supplied by this nerve. The affected muscles in spasm will hold the neck in a fixed position pulling it towards the affected side. This is medically called scoliosis or, in the neck, in particular, 'torticollis'. With the prolapsed disc in these sites, brachial neuritis never occurs, although pain may extend downwards to the base of the neck and upwards to the base of the skull with a moderate post-occipital neuritis. Unfortunately, quite often there are no noticeably particular features and often a spinal lesion here is not diagnosed, though in my opinion, most cases showing torticollis, without another apparent cause, are due to a slipped disc lesion.

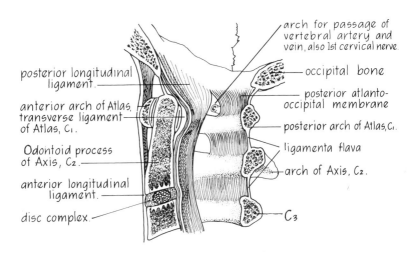

posterior longitudinal ligament.

anterior arch of Atlas, transverse ligament of Atlas, C₁.

Odontoid process of Axis, C₂.

anterior longitudinal ligament.

disc complex.

arch for passage of vertebral artery and vein, also 1st cervical nerve.

occipital bone

posterior atlanto-occipital membrane

posterior arch of Atlas,C₁.

ligamenta flava

arch of Axis, C₂.

C₃

A. (above) Schematic lateral section of the occipital bone and the first three cervical vertebrae.

B. (below) Schematic posterior veiw of the occipital bone and the first three cervical vertebrae.

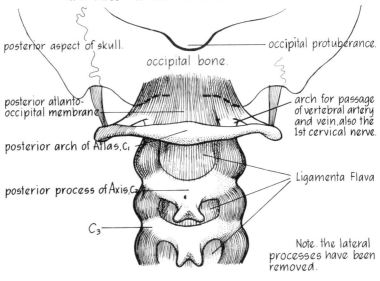

posterior aspect of skull.

occipital protuberance.

occipital bone.

posterior atlanto-occipital membrane

arch for passage of vertebral artery and vein,also the 1st cervical nerve.

posterior arch of Atlas,C₁.

Ligamenta Flava

posterior process of Axis,C₂.

C₃

Note. the lateral processes have been removed.

Diag. 53. Upper cervical ligaments.

112

3. Symptoms of a Slipped Disc Lesion between the Base of the Skull and C.1

When a disc lesion occurs at this site, admittedly rarely, the clinical picture shows a marked spasm of muscles on the affected side pulling the head slightly towards that side and, in most cases, there is also post-occipital neuritis, because the prolapsed disc is mechanically pressing on the occipital nerve root. This will give rise to pain over the back of the head on one side or the other, and sometimes even both sides may be involved. For example, if the left side is affected, the pain may continue to run right over the top of the head, causing a migraine-like syndrome, often also with pain in the left supra-orbital region, that is pain just above the left eye. A similar clinical picture will occur if the disc lesion is on the right side.

These symptoms, especially those associated with the migraine syndrome, occur not only as a result of a disc lesion at this level, for this is comparatively rare, but also as a direct result of the complicated disposition of the anatomical structures in the upper part of the cervical area.

In this region, the condyles of the base of the skull articulate with the superior aspect of C.1, which is the atlas. A small amount of annular ligament, sometimes surrounding a tiny rudimentary disc or nucleus pulposus, is present in this joint, although in most cases, this disc is completely absent. The odontoid process of the axis or C.2 emerges through a specific channel in the atlas or C.1, to articulate with the base of the skull. At this level, the spinal cord enters the skull to join up with the brain. The arteries to the brain also enter the brain through specific foramina, accompanied by their respective veins. The post-occipital nerve passing from the superior aspect of the cord, runs in close proximity to these vessels.

The post-occipital artery, accompanied by its vein and nerve, passes at each side through a static bony canal at the posterior aspect of the base of the skull, and this canal does not yield to internal pressure. If, for any reason, dilatation occurs in the artery as, for example, following excessive or prolonged forward flexion of the head, the bony canal will not yield to accommodate the dilated artery. Thus mechanical pressure is exerted on the nerve giving rise to a post-occipital neuritis (that is, headaches of varying degree) or a migraine-like syndrome. Pain may extend over the occiput, on one side or the other or even both.

Usually there is also dilatation of the supra-orbital artery. Thus pain will be present because of pressure on the supra-orbital nerve, i.e. supra-orbital neuritis. Sometimes dilatation of the infra-orbital artery also occurs giving pain in this region.

The dilated arteries may also cause compression of their accompanying veins. This disturbance of the venous flow from the brain will give rise to a moderate degree of cerebral oedema and the symptoms of this will affect vision. Patients will complain of distorted vision, spots in front of their eyes or flashes of light. Clinically, this is called 'aura'. Nausea, with an occasional accompaniment of actual vomiting, is a common symptom, depending on the severity of the cerebral congestion. All the symptoms vary considerably from patient to patient, depending on the amount of disturbance caused by the dilated arteries. This condition and its treatment is complicated and further discussion would be out of context here, and should be separately considered.

When a disc lesion is present in any of the above three different cervical areas, there is commonly an overlapping of clinical features. For example, with a disc lesion at cervical 6/7 a torticollis may be present with the pain extending upwards to the mid-neck region with a slight post-occipital neuritis. Moderate post-occipital neuritis may occur with the disc lesion in the mid cervical area. With a lesion at the superior aspect of the neck, a slight scoliosis extending downwards may be present, but at this site brachial neuritis never occurs.

The Non-Surgical Detachment of a Disc in the Cervical Region

Diagnosis

I take a very careful clinical history, particularly as regards the patient's cervical condition. If the patient is wearing, or has been using a cervical collar I advise that the collar be discarded, because such use causes disuse atrophy in the affected muscles. The patient is asked to remove his clothing from the neck, shoulders and arms and I examine the cervical area for spasm or any twisting of the neck (torticollis); spasm of the muscles over the shoulder girdle; or any degree of wasting in the intrinsic muscles of the hand. I carry out a grip test to assess the degree of weakness or otherwise of the grip. If the median or ulnar nerves are both involved then the grip of that affected side will be practically nil and this will indicate the lesion has occurred between cervical 6/7. If the grip is deficient on the thenar, or thumb side, then the median nerve is involved. If the grip is deficient on the hypothenar eminence, or ulnar side of the hand, then the ulnar nerve is involved.

I examine the patient in the erect posture with his back towards me. I place my hands on either side of the head and gently pull the head backwards, noting how far it will come without pain or any diminution of movement. I then bring the head to one side, noting again how far it will come and then bring it round to the other side.

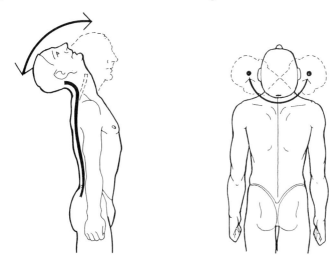

Diag. 54. Test to assess neck mobility.

The extent of movement is recorded on the patient's record card. I attempt a slight rotation of the skull through the cervical region and again assess the amount of movement without pain. Usually there is a marked loss of cervical movement in all directions. In many cases this is due to a degree of cervical spondylosis, that is, a contraction of the intrinsic ligaments and muscles of the cervical region (see chapter IX). In some cases these symptoms may be due to a slipped disc lesion, for which the treatment has included the wearing of a cervical collar. This may have allowed the intrinsic ligaments and muscles to atrophy and contract, which in turn could give rise to a marked loss of neck movement, thus simulating the clinical picture of a cervical spondylosis.

Treatment

If a slipped disc lesion is diagnosed, the treatment is to detach the slipped disc non-surgically under local anaesthesia, as described before in the previous two chapters. The disc between the cervical vertebral bodies is the easiest to treat, because the amount of muscle surrounding the neck is far, far less in volume than that of the lumbar region. Thus access to the disc complex is relatively easy.

The Treatment of Deformity in the Cervical Region by Surgical Manipulation

After the injection of local anaesthesia, and the non-surgical detachment of the disc and whilst the muscles are still flaccid, I place one hand on top of the patient's head and with the thumb of the other hand physically press straight through the area of muscle that was in spasm at the site of the lesion.

With one hand still on the top of the head, with the other hand I pull the head backwards to a degree far greater than when I originally examined the patient. I then rotate the head, still in a backward direction, bringing the head round, ear towards the shoulder, but never forwards. In other words, I am performing the round part of a capital 'D'. I continue this process from side to side about six times and in some cases audible clicks occur as one facet rubs agains the other. The spasm in the muscles which was pulling the head to one side or the other begins to relax at this stage.

The Training Programme for Cervical Disc Lesions

Muscles that are in spasm, caused by the mechanical pressure of the disc on the nerve root supplying those muscles, are usually, by definition not in good tone. Thus I therefore again prescribe an appropriate training programme to regain tone in the affected muscles. These prescribed exercises must not be neglected, for the muscles must eventually be strengthened, in this case to support the head in its normal alignment. They must be performed daily with patience and perseverance especially if the condition is longstanding. It is important that the patient takes deep breaths with each movement as oxygen is essential for muscle regeneration and toning.

This training programme is designed to regain muscle tone in the neck and supra scapular muscles, and to smooth the respective facet joints.

EXERCISE I: (Cervical)

With the patient standing erect the head is jerked backwards and forwards but only to the erect posture, i.e. never bending the neck downwards. This should be done 10 times.

Exercise I

1. Stand erect with feet together.
2. Jerk the head backwards, and then forwards but only as far as the erect posture, (never bending the neck forwards).
3. Repeat 10 times.

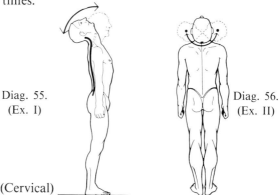

Diag. 55.
(Ex. I)

Diag. 56.
(Ex. II)

EXERCISE II: (Cervical)

With the head held backwards the patient rotates the head in this axis, the ear towards the shoulder, five times in one direction and then rotates it five times in the opposite direction, following the course of the round part of a capital 'D'. The patient is asked to avoid bringing the head forwards beyond the shoulder point.

Exercise II

1. Stand erect with feet together.
2. Hold the head backwards.
3. Rotate the head in this axis, ear to shoulder, five times to one side. Avoid bringing the head forwards beyond the shoulder point.
4. Similarly, rotate in the opposite direction five times.
5. The rotation should follow the course of the round part of a capital 'D'. The head should never be rotated round and round as this will cause dizziness.

EXERCISE III: (Cervical)

The patient keeps his head back, and looks up at the ceiling with his arms straight out in front, fists clenched, and performs a swimming motion with his arms, keeping them absolutely rigid with no bending at all at the elbows and wrists. He must keep the arms outstretched and parallel with the ground until the scapulae are almost touching, then drop the arms to the side and then bring them straight up to the erect forward position again. This should be done 20 times, four times a day.

This exercise not only gets the muscles of the neck in good tone but also the supra-scapular, medial scapular and the arm muscles. If there is a degree of cervical spondylosis present, exercises II and III — the rotation of the head in the shape of a 'D' and the "swimming" exercise — will tone up both the affected muscles and ligaments and a full range of movement will be obtained.

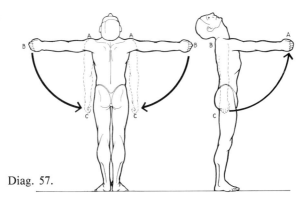

Diag. 57.

Exercise III

1. Stand erect with feet together.

2. Hold the head back, looking up to the ceiling.

3. Stretch the arms out straight in front and parallel to the floor.

4. With elbow joints fixed and fists clenched rotate the stiff arms quickly backwards as in swimming breast stroke, with the shoulder blades coming together when the arms are right back.

5. Swing the stiff arms down past the body and repeat 20 times, four times a day. Take a deep breath when the arms are being raised to the horizontal plane, and exhale as the shoulder blades are brought together.

118

EXERCISE IV: (Cervical)

The patient may do this exercise standing or sitting. Commencing with the head erect and looking forward he should turn the neck slowly but firmly sideways until the chin is in line with the top of the shoulder. Then pause for a count of three and return to the front. This should be repeated 5 times in each direction, three or four times a day.

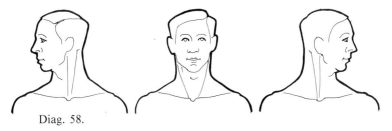

Diag. 58.

Exercise IV

1. The patient may sit or stand for this exercise.
2. With the head erect and looking forward, turn the neck slowly but firmly sideways, until the chin is in line with the top of the shoulder. Then pause for a count of five.
3. Perform the exercise five times in each direction, three or four times a day.

All these exercises should be carried out at least three or four times a day. Sportsmen and women, in particular, should carry out this programme every hour of the day until all symptoms have gone and the affected muscles are in good tone. For many of my patients, I recommend that they carry out this training programme for a minute or two, night and morning, for all time. On average, it usually takes 2-3 weeks for the condition to resolve and a full range of movement to be obtained.

There is, in time, practically no pain with a normal range of movements. The pain, at first, is simply the start of the muscles coming into action again after a disuse atrophy. On the day following the commencement of the treatment, there will be a marked increase of pain, similar to that which occurs when one has played the first game of sport at the beginning of the season, but this should settle after two or three days, and more and more freedom of movement with less and less pain will be achieved.

119

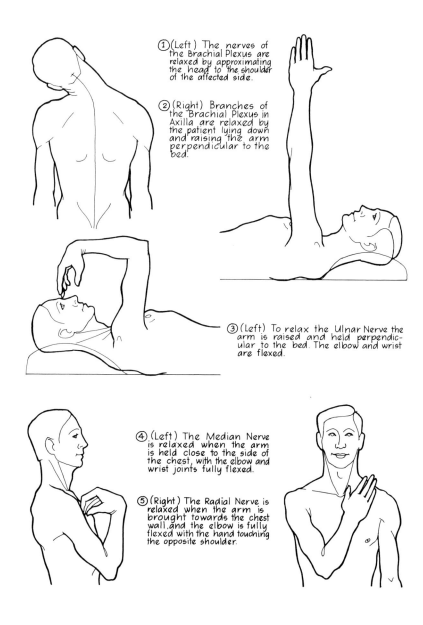

1. (Left) The nerves of the Brachial Plexus are relaxed by approximating the head to the shoulder of the affected side.

2. (Right) Branches of the Brachial Plexus in Axilla are relaxed by the patient lying down and raising the arm perpendicular to the bed.

3. (Left) To relax the Ulnar Nerve the arm is raised and held perpendicular to the bed. The elbow and wrist are flexed.

4. (Left) The Median Nerve is relaxed when the arm is held close to the side of the chest, with the elbow and wrist joints fully flexed.

5. (Right) The Radial Nerve is relaxed when the arm is brought towards the chest wall, and the elbow is fully flexed with the hand touching the opposite shoulder.

Diag. 59. Methods of relaxing the nerves of the brachial plexus.

120

It is important to avoid any state that will aggravate the condition whilst symptoms still persist. During sleep, patients are advised to try and keep the cervical column in a straight line with the remainder of the spinal column. Pillows may be placed to fill in the square between the side of the head and the shoulder, when the patient is lying on his side. If only one pillow is used in this position, the head may fall towards it, and thus aggravate the pain in the neck. If however, three pillows are used, the head may be over-flexed leading to acute strain and further pain. Usually, two pillows provide the satisfactory height. The above principle applies also when the patient is lying on his back. A small 9″ x 4″ bolster may be used to support the neck in this position. I recommend the use of down-filled pillows for all patients suffering from pain in the neck.

Patients should also avoid wearing a garment which pulls the shoulder joint downwards, as this aggravates the brachial neuritis by the downward pull of the sensitive nerve roots. For example, females should be sure to wear a correctly fitting bra. The straps of this, if

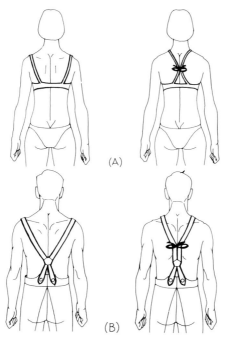

Diag. 60. Methods of alleviating brachial neuritis.

pulling on the points of the shoulder joints, should be pulled medially towards the base of the neck. This can be done by cutting the elastic straps at the back and restitching them 2″ nearer the mid-line. Another method of achieving the same result is to tie the posterior straps to one another with a short piece of tape. If male patients wear braces, pull on the points of the shoulders is prevented by fixing the anterior clips towards the mid-line, or by tying the posterior straps together with a tape.

Patients should avoid the use of the affected arm for one week, if necessary supporting it in a sling, to avoid pulling on the sensitive nerve plexus, or even easing the pull by placing the hand at intervals inside a fastened jacket. Heavy lifts should not be attempted for about three weeks.

A surgical collar must never be worn as this leads to disuse atrophy in the neck muscles. Some patients wearing one suffer from a choking feeling and some from claustrophobia.

Coughing or sneezing must be avoided as far as possible. These cause a wave pressure of the cerebro-spinal fluid that surrounds the brain and the whole of the spinal cord. This wave will strike the hypersensitive affected nerve root and cause sharp sudden intense pain.

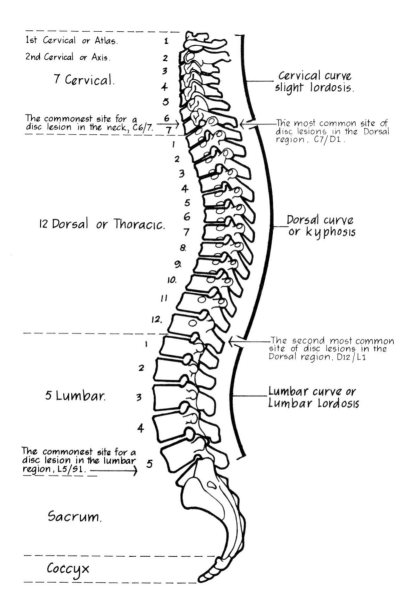

1st Cervical or Atlas. **1**

2nd Cervical or Axis. **2**

3

7 Cervical. **4**

5

The commonest site for a disc lesion in the neck, C6/7. **6** → **7** ← The most common site of disc lesions in the Dorsal region, C7/D1.

Cervical curve slight lordosis.

I

2

3

4

5

6

12 Dorsal or Thoracic. **7**

8.

9.

10.

11

12.

Dorsal curve or kyphosis

← The second most common site of disc lesions in the Dorsal region, D12/L1

1

2

5 Lumbar. **3**

Lumbar curve or Lumbar Lordosis

4

The commonest site for a disc lesion in the lumbar region, L5/S1. ——→ **5**

Sacrum.

Coccyx

Diag. 61. Lateral view of the spinal column showing the commonest sites for disc lesions in the dorsal region.

124

Diagnosis and Treatment of a Slipped Disc Lesion in the Dorsal (Thoracic) Region

THE DORSAL area of the spinal column consists of twelve vertebrae, the first dorsal articulating with the 7th cervical, and the twelfth dorsal vertebra articulating with the first lumbar, in each case through the mutual annular ligament intervening. These two extremes of the dorsal region are the commonest sites of the slipped disc lesion of the dorsal area; the one is closest to the neck where there is a great deal of movement and the other to the pelvis where there is a moderate range of movement. As in all disc lesions, injury, i.e. trauma, is the essential cause, which leads to a tear in the annular ligament and the prolapsing disc striking a nerve root. Acute pain will occur at the affected site with a moderate degree of muscle spasm, leading to a moderate degree of scoliosis at the affected level. Prolapsed discs are not common between these two sites as there is very little movement of the vertebrae which are further stabilised by the articulation with the ribs, However, they do occur, and sudden injury plays a vital role. They are usually the results of accidents, such as a motor crash, or a collapse of a rugby scrum. From a clinical point of view the disc lesion conditions in the dorsal area may be divided into three regions:

1. Disc lesions between C.7/D.1

2. Disc lesions between D.2/3, 3/4, 4/5, 5/6, 6/7, 7/8, 8/9, 9/10, 10/11 and 11/12

3. Disc lesions between D.12/L.1.

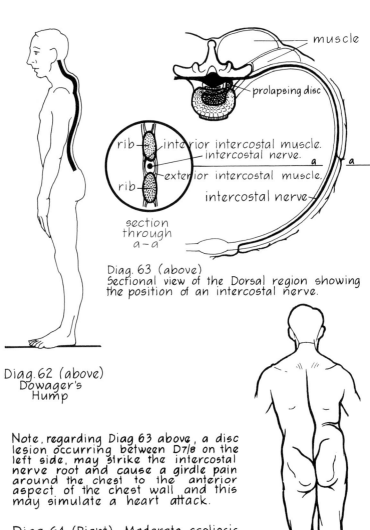

muscle

prolapsing disc

rib — interior intercostal muscle.
— intercostal nerve.

exterior intercostal muscle.

intercostal nerve

rib

section
through
a–a

Diag. 63 (above)
Sectional view of the Dorsal region showing
the position of an intercostal nerve.

Diag. 62 (above)
   Dowager's
   Hump

Note, regarding Diag 63 above, a disc
lesion occurring between D7/8 on the
left side, may strike the intercostal
nerve root and cause a girdle pain
around the chest to the anterior
aspect of the chest wall and this
may simulate a heart attack.

Diag 64 (Right). Moderate scoliosis
caused by a disc lesion in the Dorsal
area at D12/L1, occurs at a higher level
than that caused by a disc lesion in
the lumbar area.

Diags. 62, 63 and 64. Conditions arising from
    disc lesions in the dorsal area.

126

1. **Symptoms of a Disc Lesion between C.7/D.1.**

This is the most common site of a disc lesion in the dorsal part of the spinal column as most movement occurs here. Acute pain is usually felt at the base of the neck on the affected side. The muscles at this level go into spasm, pulling the spinal column towards them. This scoliosis is usually very slight. Pain may be referred into the supra scapular group of muscles and, at times, down the medial scapular muscles to the lower aspect of the scapula. It is extremely rare to get brachial involvement with a lesion in this area. A common feature is flattening of the normal cervical lordosis due to the pull of the post-cervical muscles going into spasm. At times a complete reversal of the cervical lordosis may arise. In very severe cases there is a marked prominence of the posterior processes of C.5/6/7 and D.1/2, giving rise to a moderate degree of **'Dowager's Hump'** (see also Chapter IX).

2. **Symptoms of a Disc Lesion between D.2/3, 3/4, 4/5, 5/6, 6/7, 7/8, 8/9, 9/10 and 10/11**

Prolapsed discs may occur in the dorsal region between the above mentioned two most usual sites. However, as a rule, these only occur when a severe blow or injury has been sustained, and consequently, it is quite common to have also a fracture of an adjacent rib where it articulates with the vertebra. A disc lesion occurring, admittedly rarely, between D.7/8 can give rise to girdle pain round the chest to the anterior chest wall, which, if it is on the left side, may simulate a heart attack. If there is the slightest doubt in these cases, an electro-cardiograph is carried out.

3. **Symptoms of a Disc Lesion Between D.12 and L.1.**

This is the second most common site for a disc lesion in the thoracic region. Acute pain is usually felt at the site of the prolapsed disc. Marked spasm of muscles will lead to a moderate degree of scoliosis. Referred pain may occur in the anterior lower aspect of the abdominal wall which, on the right side, may clinically give the features of an acute appendicitis or renal colic.

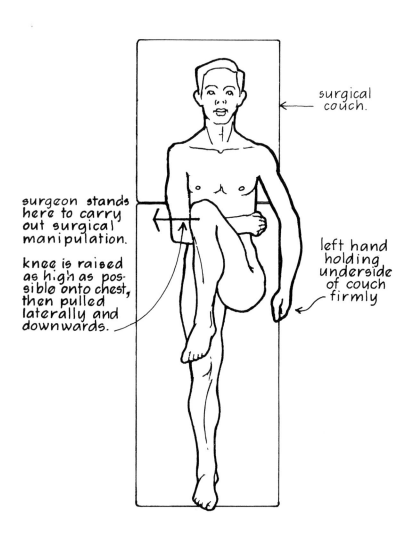

surgical couch.

surgeon stands here to carry out surgical manipulation.

knee is raised as high as possible onto chest, then pulled laterally and downwards.

left hand holding underside of couch firmly

Diag. 65. Surgical manipulation for dorsal disc lesions.

128

The Non-Surgical Detachment of a Disc
in the Dorsal Region

The dorsal disc lesion is the most difficult to treat by the non-surgical detachment technique. The ribs articulate with the vertebrae and this prevents one from getting clearly to the disc and detaching it. However, it can be done and is carried out in a similar manner to that of the cervical or lumbar disc lesions.

If a mid-dorsal lesion is being treated on, for example, the left side, the patient is asked to put his left hand down on the right knee and remain in that position. Then I rotate the chest. Thus the dorsal vertebral bodies and lateral processes, in particular, are separated and, in that way, I can inject the local anaesthetic into the nerve root and then go ahead with the non-surgical detachment of the disc described in detail in chapters IV and V. Corresponding treatment is given for a disc lesion on the right side.

Treatment of the Deformity in the Dorsal Region
by Surgical Manipulation

The patient is asked to lie flat on his back on the surgical couch with the affected segment of his spinal column towards me. As in manipulation of the lumbar lesions, the knee on the unaffected side is bent upwards towards the chest, and if possible, in these dorsal lesion cases, the knee is brought up close to the chest wall. This permits flexion of the dorsal spinal column. The patient's hand on the unaffected side holds on to the underside of the couch. I then bend this flexed knee joint towards myself with one hand, whilst the other hand is placed on the unaffected part of the dorsal spinal column. I gently pull the limb towards me and point it towards the unaffected shoulder joint. As a rule, there may be an audible click which is due to one facet clicking over the other. The limb is pulled downwards, but still remains pointing towards the shoulder joint until the deformity of the dorsal spinal column is corrected. Usually 3 or 4 'surgical' manipulations are required.

The Training Programme for Dorsal Disc Lesions

As usual, I prescribe a training programme to regain tone in the affected muscles. The prescribed exercises must not be neglected but be performed daily with patience and perseverance especially if the condition is longstanding. The muscles must be strengthened to support the spinal column in its normal alignment. It must be remembered that muscles will quickly lose their tone if they are not kept active, and that oxygen is essential for muscle building, so deep breaths must be taken when performing the exercises.

EXERCISE I: (Dorsal)

The patient stands perfectly erect with the arms held like rods laterally, parallel with the floor and fists kept clenched. The patient then quickly whips the arms from side to side, which moves the dorsal part of the spine. The exercise should be done four times a day, 20 movements in each direction. The feet must be kept firmly on the ground.

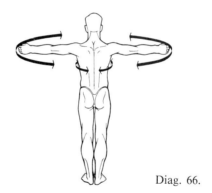

Diag. 66.

Exercise I

1. Stand in the erect posture, with feet together.
2. With stiff elbow and wrist joints and clenched fists stretch the arms out sideways at shoulder level, parallel to the floor.
3. Rotate the chest as far as it will go, from side to side. This, in turn, rotates the dorsal or thoracic vertebrae.
4. Repeat 20 times in each direction four times a day.
5. Breathe in and out with each movement.

130

EXERCISE II: (Dorsal)

The patient stands with his arms stretched out like rods, at shoulder level with fists clenched. He then lowers one arm, and raises the other by bending at the waistline, still making sure that the arms are kept straight and in line with the tip of the shoulders. Holding this posture he whips the arms first one way and then the other, 20 times in each direction. This exercise should be repeated 20 further times with the chest flexed at the waist in the opposite direction.

This exercise quickly gets into action those muscles that had lost their tone. Also the rotating movement involved allows more disc to protrude through the tear in the annular ligament, the sharp edges of which will usually automatically cut off this protruding disc.

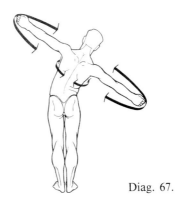

Diag. 67.

Exercise II

1. Stand in the erect posture with feet together.
2. With stiff elbows and wrist joints and clenched fists stretch the arms out sideways at shoulder level, parallel to the floor.
3. Lower one arm, bending at the waist with the other pointing upwards, still with the arm straight and in line with the tip of the shoulders.
4. Holding this posture, whip the arms first one way and then the other.
5. Repeat 20 times in each direction.
6. Repeat 20 further times with the chest flexed at the waist in the opposite direction.
7. Inhale and exhale regularly to prevent overtiring of the muscles.

EXERCISE III: (Dorsal)

This exercise can be carried out sitting or standing, and has the effect of muscle toning traction. The patient clasps his hands on top of his head and the elbows are raised as high as possible laterally. He then swings the chest from side to side for about 2″ inches, extending himself upwards with every movement, 20 times to each side.

Exercise III (Diag. 68)

1. The patient may either sit or stand.
2. Clasp hands on the top of the head, with elbows raised as high as possible.
3. Swing the chest from side to side for about 2″, extending upwards with every movement.
4. Repeat 20 times in each direction.

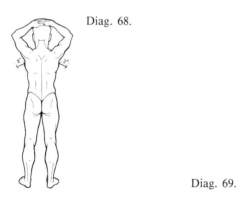

Diag. 68.

Diag. 69.

EXERCISE IV: (Dorsal)

In the same posture, rotation may be carried out, 2″ in all directions, again 20 times in each direction.

Exercise IV (Diag. 69)

1. Adopt the same posture as for Exercise III.
2. Rotate the chest, bending 2″ in all directions.
3. Repeat 20 times one way, and 20 times the other.

If the patient follows this training programme, he is helping me to help himself get fit and he is usually cured after 10-14 days. However, in some cases (about 2-3%) symptoms can be slow to clear depending, possibly, on the length of time the patient has been suffering. Also, in older age groups, a patient's symptoms are somewhat slower to clear up.

It helps if the patient understands why the pain persists in some cases. When a slipped disc has been striking a nerve root for a considerable time the nerve will have become very, very sensitive and may remain so for some time after the striking has been discontinued. This is similar to the way in which the pain from a blow on the chin will last much longer than the actual blow and the injured area will remain sensitive for some considerable time.

Patients are asked to avoid stooping and toe touching as this only aggravates the condition. Heavy lifting should also be avoided. When sitting or standing and indeed walking, they should maintain as far as possible the erect posture. They should preferably sit in a relatively 'upright' sprung-backed chair so that the dorsal part of the spinal column is held erect and supported along its whole length. The usual type of very soft easy chair or couches should be avoided because they are usually too low and too deep to give proper back support. The actual length of the seat cushion is usually too long for the length of the average human thigh. From an orthopaedic point of view, I would advise furnishing manufacturers to consider decreasing the seat depth and increasing the seat height of their easy chairs and couches. This would be of great benefit to those who suffer from a back problem, and are seeking chairs with good back support, to get relief from pain or discomfort. (See diagram overleaf).

Quick jerky movements should be avoided and all forms of sport discontinued for 2-3 weeks. Diving should be avoided, although swimming is an excellent exercise for this condition. The patient will find that deep breathing will aggravate the discomfort but shallow breathing will minimise the movement of the ribs at the site of the disc lesion.

Patients will find it more comfortable to rest on a good interior sprung mattress and should avoid a hardboard bed, lying always on the unaffected side.

Coughing or sneezing should be avoided as they cause a wave of pressure of the cerebro-spinal fluid that surrounds the brain and the whole of the spinal cord. This wave will strike the hypersensitive affected nerve root and cause sharp sudden intense pain.

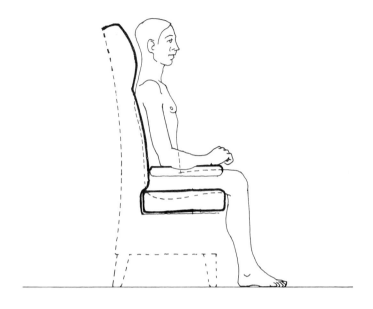

① The chair should be relatively upright with a well sprung back, to support the contour of the whole spinal column. It should also have a relatively high seat.

② To obtain relief from lower back pain, patients should sit with their buttocks into the back of the seat and their feet on the floor. They should also ensure that the thighs are at right angles to the leg and that the seat cushion causes no pressure behind the knee joints.

③ Most seat cushions of easy chairs and couches are too deep for the length of the adult thigh, and often the seats are too low. These two factors, especially in combination, mean that the individual has great difficulty in regaining the erect posture.

Diag. 70. Recommended posture requirements for easy chairs.

134

CHAPTER VIII

An Analysis of Other Known Methods of Treatment with a Qualified Opinion as to the Value or Otherwise of Each

INJURIES TO the intravertebral disc complex present a comparatively new clinical entity and this may account for no diagnosis, or incorrect diagnosis, being given in the past. It is only within recent years that the symptoms of the slipped disc lesion have been fully understood, and recognised. Even so, the clinical picture is, at times, difficult to differentiate from other causes of pain in the affected area of the back. These may be nothing more than a simple strain or sprain of the articular ligaments, joint capsules or muscle attachments of the spinal column. Even after suffering an accident involving whiplash injury to the spinal column, the patient may suffer nothing more than a strain or sprain in the spinal ligaments or overstretching of the facet joint capsules. The patient's own doctor in such cases will prescribe an analgesic (i.e. a simple pain killing drug) and recommend complete rest of the affected area for a few days. Occasionally, a rubefacient (or rub) may be prescribed to help to relieve the muscle spasm and so diminish the pain. The pain, whether in the lumbar area or the cervical, usually clears up in three or four days.

If, however, the patient after an accident or at the time of consultation, shows neurological symptoms, e.g. brachial neuritis involving pain in the cervical area, or sciatica after injury to the lower lumbar region, then these cases require further investigation in the Neuro- or Orthopaedic departments in a hospital to diagnose or exclude a slipped disc lesion condition.

135

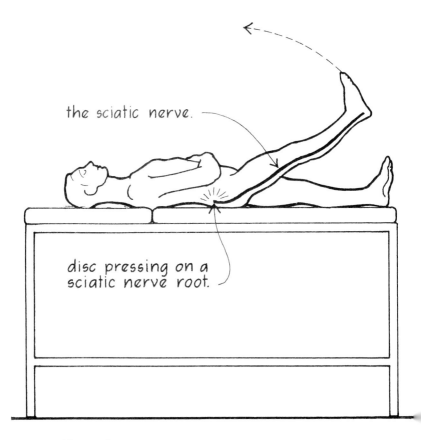

the sciatic nerve.

disc pressing on a
sciatic nerve root.

The whole sciatic nerve is hypersensitive.
Thus by carrying out the straight leg
raising test one is stretching the nerve
thereby increasing the sciatica.

This test should be avoided.

Diag. 71. Straight leg raising test.

I should like to discuss a number of current methods of diagnosis and treatment of slipped disc lesions which seem to me either to treat only the symptoms, or are not wholly successful even after painful treatment, perhaps even involving surgery. It seems that almost each consultant has his, or her, own method of dealing with the same type of clinical condition and this must surely suggest that there is no clear answer to the medical problem involved. I maintain that a complete cure can only be effected if the cause of the pain is eradicated. The root cause of all the pain in slipped disc lesions is the physical striking of the prolapsed disc on to the nerve root and thus the disc must be detached to get rid of all the symptoms permanently.

The following is a list of the current methods of diagnosis and treatment and I will try to explain why, in my opinion, these methods are often of uncertain value.

1. Diagnosis Using Straight Leg Raising Test

Most doctors and orthopaedic consultants include this technique as part of the routine examination for the slipped disc condition in the lumbar area with sciatica. The patient is asked to lie prone on the surgical couch and raise the leg at the affected side. The consultant monitors the ease with which the patient raises the leg and the height to which he can raise it by himself, and also with the doctor's assistance. This manoeuvre stretches the already hypersensitive sciatic nerve which is already causing the patient great pain.

It seems to me that it is an unfortunate medical practice that, in order only to confirm a diagnosis, one should actually aggravate the condition one is about to try and clear up. I have, in previous chapters, described the symptoms in detail of slipped discs in each area of the spinal column and an assessment of these symptoms will in each case, I believe, lead to a confident diagnosis. The obvious confirmation of sciatica is the absence of ankle reflex that can easily and painlessly be tested. The patient's description of the pain will normally show the picture of the nerve tract, the root of which is being struck by the slipped disc, despite the fact that the patient may often have no detailed anatomical knowledge. After the patient's description of his symptoms, the consultant can proceed to a more detailed examination and from this come to a firm diagnosis without causing the patient more distress and pain. The non-surgical detachment of disc that I advocate leads to complete cure within 14 days in 90% of cases and certainly eliminates the excruciating 'nerve'

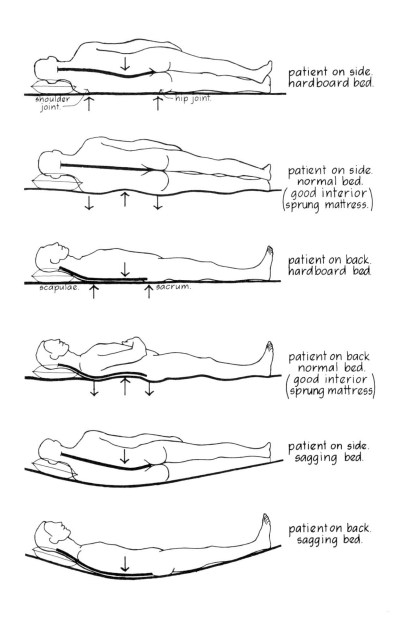

patient on side.
hardboard bed.

shoulder joint. hip joint.

patient on side.
normal bed.
(good interior sprung mattress.)

patient on back.
hardboard bed.

scapulae. sacrum.

patient on back.
normal bed.
(good interior sprung mattress)

patient on side.
sagging bed.

patient on back.
sagging bed.

Diag. 72. Sleeping postures.

138

pain. In my opinion, monitoring by means of this leg raising test during treatment is also unnecessary and painful. It actually painfully retards the progress, for it causes the still sensitive nerve to be stretched once again.

2. The Orthopaedic Bed or Bed with Hardboard Underneath

Many patients are advised to lie on a hard bed for 6-8 weeks. Bedding manufacturers have produced these so-called 'orthopaedic beds' to simulate the hardness and flatness attained by placing a sheet of hardboard under a firm mattress. I personally deplore this form of therapy and consider the term 'orthopaedic' wrongly applied to these beds. The term 'orthopaedic' simply means the correction of a deformity and in my opinion the orthopaedic bed not only does not correct, but actually aggravates the condition.

Anatomically the body is not designed to lie on a hard flat surface. Even in the army I noticed young and fit soldiers asking for help to get up after sleeping on the hard ground all night. Thus if perfectly healthy young men find sleeping on a hard surface intolerable, it seems inconceivable that similar conditions would prove beneficial to a back sufferer. My experience has been that, in almost every case of a painful back, lying on a hard surface has only aggravated the condition.

Most back patients prefer to sleep on their sides or back. If the patient lies on his side on a hard bed, the bony prominences of his shoulder and the hip bone are held fixed and the remainder of his lumbar area extending up towards the dorsal aspect of the spine, sags unsupported downwards to the hard surface. If, however, the patient lies on a good interior sprung mattress the bony prominences of the shoulder, hip and pelvic area are impaled into the softness of the bed and between these points the mattress forms a bulge which gives support for the affected lumbar area of the spinal column. Similarly, when the patient lies on his back on a hard flat bed, the posterior aspect of the upper dorsal, i.e. the scapular region, forms one fixed point, and the posterior aspect of the pelvis forms the other. Thus the area of the spinal column between these two points of the back is left unsupported (see diagram).

Treatment which entails lying on a hard bed for 6-8 weeks is rarely effective and is also very frustrating for the average patient. Few men can spend six weeks away from work and mothers of young children equally find it impracticable to lie in bed for a lengthy period without outside help in the home. In a few cases the condition does settle down after prolonged rest. The disc may move off the nerve either due to atrophy in rare cases, or rotation of the spinal column. However, in the latter case, even a little cough or sneeze can cause the symptoms to recur, if the disc has, for instance, reverted into a position where it is again striking the nerve root.

3. The Use of Plaster Casts, Surgical Corsets and Cervical Collars

In an attempt to immobilise the patient's spinal column, and still permit mobility, the consultant often recommends a corset, cervical collar or plaster cast. The latter is uncomfortable and distressing to the wearer and often gives him a sense of claustrophobia. The corset may be elasticated, thus fitting a range of body shapes and so available "off the shelf", but more often a surgical one is recommended and is carefully measured and made up for the patient. In this case, obviously, a delay is caused before treatment can commence. However, the main disadvantage of these methods is that, in order to immobilise the spinal column, the muscles which are in spasm, as a result of disc lesion with scoliosis, and whose job it is to control the movements of the column, are also immobilised. If no movement is allowed (or even very restricted movement), these muscles soon develop what we call, clinically, a disuse atrophy. This is demonstrated clearly when, after a broken limb has been encased in plaster for two or three weeks, the limb becomes literally only skin and bone. This shows just how rapidly disuse atrophy sets into muscles not in action, whether they are in spasm or not. Similarly, by preventing movement by means of any spinal support or cervical collar a massive atrophy can, and does, set into the spinal muscles between the vertebrae, i.e. the intrinsic muscles. I, therefore, deplore the use of these supports and, for these reasons, would never recommend their use for the disc lesion condition.

4. Physiotherapy and Exercises

In order to avoid muscle atrophy caused either, by lying up for 6-8 weeks or through wearing a support, the patient will often be given treatment by a physiotherapist. Physiotherapy is a very valuable method of dealing with muscles out of tone or with joints that require gentle manipulation. However, in the case of the slipped disc the physiotherapist would be dealing only with the outward symptoms of the complaint. The muscles are in spasm because of the compressed nerve roots and exercise of these spastic muscles only gives further pain and may cause secondary symptoms, such as spinal deformity. The muscle cannot regenerate as long as the nerve supply is being interfered with by the disc pressure. I recommend wholeheartedly the use of exercises and prescribe a complete training programme to bring the muscles back into tone but only after treatment to detach the disc has begun, and the muscles are becoming relaxed and out of spasm,

Physiotheraphy is of great value once the disc has been detached. Then heat treatment, massage and electrical muscle stimulation are most helpful.

Various types of electrical apparatus have been evolved in order to give **electrical stimulation** to the affected muscles which are in acute spasm and causing pain. This treatment, in my opinion, may only give temporary relief as the cause of the patient's symptoms, which is the presence of the prolapsed disc striking a nerve root, is still present.

5. Traction

When undergoing this form of treatment the patient lies on a 'hardboard' bed and heavy weights are attached to his feet in such a way as to exert a pull on the spinal column in an attempt to separate the vertebral bodies and so, in theory, alleviate the pressure of the disc on the affected nerve root. In some cases, fixed traction is applied where the patient is literally put on to a rack with a fixture under the arms and another fixture on to the feet and the whole body is pulled apart. I suggest that, when traction is applied to the column, it is like stretching a piece of elastic. Once you have stretched it out, in a straight plane, and let it go, it invariably releases back into exactly the same position, and the treatment is thus unsuccessful in most cases. Traction is a most uncomfortable experience and most patients rebel against it.

6. Manipulation

Until quite recently this was not widely practised or advocated by consultants in the medical profession for the treatment of a disc lesion. It is, however, commonly practised by osteopaths, chiropractors and often totally unqualified 'bone-setters'. The latter, however, skilful, have not the anatomical knowledge to ensure that no harm will come as a result of their own, often severe, manipulation. Nevertheless, the treatment by all these manipulators can, at times, give relief to the patient. This ensures their popularity, for people will recommend others to them and whilst they have willing patients their practices will flourish. Their popularity has also, in a way, been caused by the distressing lack of success in curing back problems by the medical practitioner. A patient in a severe or even crippling condition will seek help from any source, however unlikely or unqualified. During my diagnosis I always enquire if the patient has been to a qualified or unqualified manipulator, as the methods employed in such cases may have been quite severe. The manipulator usually rotates the patient's pelvis. In so doing, if a disc lesion is present, the disc may be rotated off the nerve and the pain will disappear. Unfortunately, a sudden movement, a cough, sneeze or even a sudden stoop to tie a shoe lace can bring the disc back on to the nerve and the condition will have returned.

'Surgical' manipulation forms a major part of my treatment (see page 76) but only after the prolapsed disc has been detached by my non-surgical method. Disc lesions frequently cause a lateral curvature of the spinal column (scoliosis) and 'surgical' manipulation will help to straighten the column. Scoliosis can occur without a slipped disc lesion and in most of these cases x-ray will reveal a congenital deformity of the facet joints. 'Surgical' manipulation will also help to correct the resulting conditions (see Chapter IX) and a prescribed course of vigorous training is usually recommended.

The manipulator may often suggest the clicking noises during manipulation imply that the 'disc' has been 'put back' but this is a misconception. It is simply the noise of one facet clicking over another. After all, the disc is made up of a jelly-like substance and therefore cannot produce a clicking noise.

Recently, manipulation has become more accepted by the medical profession and some surgeons have tried manipulation under general anaesthetic. I question the wisdom of this approach. In such a situation the whole spinal column of the patient is flaccid, i.e. the muscles are completely relaxed, and thus there is movement in all directions. In such circumstances, it is possible for the surgeon to overstretch and even tear the muscles and ligaments, and thus aggravate the condition considerably. He may even overstretch the nerve roots and possibly seriously damage the cord itself.

7. Epidural Injections

These are carried out by some medical practitioners, but they only give temporary relief in most cases and do not affect the vital cause of the painful condition, which is due to the mechanical pressure of disc on the affected nerve root.

8. Acupuncture

The practice of acupuncture in slipped disc lesions has been proved to be totally unsuccessful. Acupuncture may, and possibly has, some value for other conditions but I repeat it is of no value whatsoever in the treatment of a slipped disc lesion, apart from a temporary alleviation of the pain involved.

9. Analgesic Drugs and Heat Treatment

Pills or capsules are produced by almost every Pharmaceutical company, with as many names, to alleviate pain. This form of medication can basically act in two ways. It may pass straight to the painful area and thus diminish the pain, or it may act on the pain centre in the brain. Some are formulated to perform the dual role. Those that pass straight to the brain may cause mental confusion and I find it difficult to obtain a clear clinical picture from a patient in this condition. Prescribed from time to time, are the so-called muscle relaxant pills, such as Valium or Librium etc. Occasionally, the patient may become addicted to such drugs and need specialised help for this condition. In any case all analgesic drugs act only temporarily by masking the pain for a short time. The pain will continue to return until the nerve root is freed from the pressure of the disc.

Sometimes injections of morphia or pethadine, even a local anaesthetic, may be necessary to alleviate temporarily acute suffering but they do not effect a cure.

The use of **Ethyl Chloride Spray** following a sprain to a joint or to a painful area in a muscle is most valuable but gives only temporary relief to the sufferer of a slipped disc. Similarly a **hot water bottle** or a **Belladonna Plaster** may help a strained muscle or a sprain of the lumbar facet joints but it cannot cure the disc lesion. The use of an **Infra Red Lamp** seems, in fact, to aggravate the condition, for it leads to a swelling of the spinal disc itself.

143

10. Cortisone Injections

A relatively recent treatment is the injection of steroids into the area of muscle spasm. This again does not attack the root cause of the trouble and it has many adverse side effects. I have never used the drug for these reasons.

11. Injections to Dissolve the Disc

Within recent times this new method has been carried out. The principle is to inject a substance into the disc hoping that this chemical will clear the problem up by dissolving the disc. In theory, this would appear to be a worthwhile method of treatment but, in practice, it is not successful. The needle used must be long and robust particularly in the lumbar region and the injection very accurately placed. As the disc and annular ligament, which surrounds it, are both developed from the notochord, if the injection can dissolve the disc, it may also affect the annular ligament and lead to all sorts of complications such as the collapse of one vertebral body onto the other. This, in turn, could affect the nerve roots and possibly lead to compression of the spinal cord.

12. Injection to Produce a Fibrosis of the Disc Itself

This is another comparatively new method of treating a slipped disc. It consists of injecting a sclerosing fluid into the disc, in order to make it firm, immobile and inert. The greatest drawback of this method is the fact that one has to use a very long needle and, in all cases, any inaccuracy could cause damage to surrounding tissues. Some who employ this method do so by making an open incision to explore the disc area. They detach only that portion of the disc which is protruding through the torn annular ligament and then inject this sclerosing fluid into the remaining portion of the disc. This method has still to be proven but it does have the advantage that laminectomy is not required and damage to nerve roots cannot readily occur, as is possible by the more usual surgical method.

13. The Cutting of Superficial Nerve Tracts

This gives only temporary relief and the results are permanent and irreversible. After all, one is cutting a nerve that may supply an area of skin or underlying muscles and the result may be permanently harmful.

14. **Surgery**

Surgery for the removal of the spinal disc is generally considered only as a last resort. Surgeons will usually admit the chances of full recovery are 50-50, for it is major surgery.

I am of the opinion that the number of good results is far lower than 50% and the risk of damage to nerves or even the spinal cord, with possible resulting paralysis, is fairly high. It is not surprising that many patients decide not to have the operation. I think it is almost tragic if an international athlete, footballer, rugby player, golfer, ballet dancer or tennis player is obliged to have an operation for, in most cases, that would be the end of his, or her, great career as a top-grade athlete. A great sportsman or woman would be lost, for even if such people were able to participate in their sport, they would never again reach the peak of their prowess. I have treated many sportsmen and sportswomen with the technique of the non-surgical detachment of the spinal disc and not only have I effected a permanent cure but, in most cases, they have continued playing their sport after two weeks of treatment. The treatment of this particular group of patients has given me a tremendous amount of personal satisfaction combining, as it does, my medical skills with my enthusiasm for sport.

Usually, the surgical procedure is laminectomy, which weakens the spinal column. The surgeon then gouges out the nucleus pulposus, i.e. disc. This actually supports my own theory that the disc is not an essential part of one's anatomy. After the removal of the disc many surgeons carry out a bone graft in order to stabilise and thus prevent movement between the opposing vertebrae at the site of operation. As with all other bone grafts the opposing bones may fail to unite and there is also a pre-disposition of the bone graft to fracture following even a mild injury, such as a slip or a sudden jerk caused by a motor car accident. If the bone graft is completely successful the opposing vertebrae are immobilised and thus a patient will always have complete loss of movement in this area.

The practice of bone grafting in slipped spinal disc lesions is, in my opinion, rather a major procedure with many inherent failure factors and, in many cases, it has proved unsuccessful. In recent years a new surgical approach for disc removal is being carried out, i.e. by the anterior or lateral approach to the affected disc. In theory, this method has many advantages. I have assessed this approach in a lot of cases, but still have not, as yet, come to a final conclusion for or against it.

15. **Disc Replacement**

Another surgical technique is to replace the disc with a nylon disc. I disapprove of this. The new disc, whether nylon or of other material, is a foreign body and may react as such. If the patient is involved in an accident the nylon disc may prolapse backwards and seriously damage the spinal cord.

Summary

A patient may have undergone many, if not all, of these treatments. He may even have been sent to a psychiatrist if the x-ray result was negative and his doctor feels the pain may be psychosomatic. What an indictment of the medical profession: that a patient be sent to a psychiatrist when he may be suffering from a physical disability! This state of affairs made me strive to perfect my own technique of the non-surgical detachment of the spinal disc under local anaesthesia, that is nerve root block. I am convinced this gives the best results and if this were not so, I would still be working in the research department for another method, and, being a surgeon, perhaps turning to a new surgical approach.

CHAPTER IX

Other Causes of Painful Back Conditions and their Treatment

THERE ARE many causes of back trouble other than the condition of a slipped disc. In order to diagnose any particular condition precisely, it is vital to be able to recognise and differentiate between the various possible conditions. Some of them show very similar symptoms to those of a slipped disc, and some are the secondary results of these, when a further congenital weakness is present.

I shall concentrate on these closely related conditions, for although I regularly treat patients suffering from still other back conditions, such as osteoporosis and varying forms of arthritis, a description of such diagnoses and the treatment involved would warrant more space than this book affords.

1. Scoliosis

Scoliosis is a condition which shows lateral curvature of the spinal column. It is a deformity of the trunk characterised by a deviation of one or more vertebrae of the spinal column from the mid-line of the body and this deviation is invariably accompanied by some degree of rotation. Scoliosis may be due to a variety of conditions.

As we have noted in a previous chapter, it is very often a direct result of a slipped disc lesion, in which case the nerve root has become compressed as a result of the slipped disc continuously striking it; the compressed nerve root has caused the muscles supplied by that nerve to go into spasm and consequently the spinal column has been pulled towards them on the affected side. This, if it occurs in the lumbar region, often produces a tilted pelvis leading to an apparent shortening of the lower limb on the affected side. Once the condition

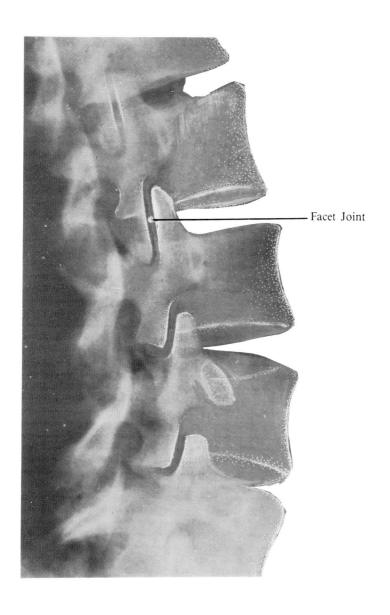

Facet Joint

Diag. 73. Photograph of an X-ray plate showing facet joints articulating in an almost vertical plane.

is cleared, up the pelvis will assume its horizontal position, and the lower limbs will again appear of equal length (see pages 27 and 87).

On the other hand, however, scoliosis may be due to congenital deformities of the spine or of the lower limbs. It can also be caused by paralysis of the muscles on one side of the column, in which case the muscles on the unaffected side pull the spinal column to that side. Other causes include injuries to the vertebral bodies, dystrophies of the skeleton and disease of the spinal ligaments or vertebrae. Adolescent Scoliosis, a congenital deformity, is a fairly common condition, and is usually recognised at an early age. Scoliosis may simply be the result of habitual faulty posture occasioned by particular duties: for example, repetitive daily work, necessitating, for instance, the carrying of heavy weights in one hand, particularly if undertaken in adolescence. Thus it is vitally important to work out a complete differential diagnosis before treatment.

Treatment

Treatment usually includes manipulation as described earlier, followed by a strict training programme to tone up the muscles affected (see pages 95-102).

2. Facet Displacement

Another condition that shows the clinical picture of a slipped disc lesion, including a marked scoliosis and sciatica is a facet displacement or subluxation. This condition, together with a detailed description of the facet joints is given in Chapter I, but because this condition has often been mis-diagnosed as a slipped disc lesion it is worth summarising it here (see page 33).

The clinical features of this type of injury may be acute pain in the lower lumbar region, over the site of the misplaced facet, and if a nerve root is struck or distorted, there may be a scoliosis and typical sciatica right down the whole length of this nerve to the foot. In some cases a bilateral sciatica may be present with acute lumbago across the lower lumbar region and possible scoliosis to one side or the other, for the side with the greater muscle spasm will pull the spinal column towards it. The diagnosis of this condition can only be confirmed by x-ray, but the radiologist must be asked for a special plate to show the facets in the affected area. The x-ray must be taken with the patient in the erect posture.

The diagnosis will usually confirm a vertical facet alignment. This usually occurs where the upper aspect of the sacrum articulates with the inferior aspect of the lumbar 5 vertebral body. Normally, the sacrum, itself formed from 5 vertebral bodies fused together to form a triangular-shaped bony mass, has its two superior facets facing backwards and inwards, but the articular facets, at this site, that is in the lumbo-sacral joints, can show great variation in their shape and the plane of their articular surfaces. For example, in the same patient the articular facets on one side may be predominantly in the horizontal plane and on the other side be predominantly in the vertical plane. If the normal anatomy of that individual has the one facet predominantly in the vertical plane, a partial dislocation of the joint can fairly easily occur: that is the inferior facet of L.5 may slip downward past the superior facet of S.1. There is a tendency for this condition to occur when the patient suffers a severe blow on the top of the head, or lands heavily on his feet or buttocks, thereby increasing a sharp forward angulation of the joint L.5/S.1. When the facets are dislocated in this way, there is usually a marked bulging of the annular ligament as the two opposing vertebral bodies come close together, and this bulging ligament may then strike a nerve root, simulating a slipped disc lesion. The fifth lumbar nerve passes through a bony canal which is directed forwards and outwards. Any distortion of the structure which goes to form the canal through which the nerve passes, can give rise to a sciatica.

In this condition, the sciatica and scoliosis are present but the diagnosis is not that of a slipped disc lesion, but that of a partial dislocation of a facet joint, the cause being inherent in the particular anatomy of that individual.

Treatment

Treatment is again mostly manipulation plus a rigorous course of training exercises to tone up the muscles that should thereafter hold the vertebrae in their correct position (see pages 95-102).

3. Ligament Strains and Sprains

The Strain of the Ligamenta Flava

This structure is made up of sections of elastic tissue attached to, and extending between the adjacent portions of the arches of the vertebrae. Its detailed anatomy is given in Appendix I, page 177.

Its essential function is that it assists in maintaining or regaining the erect posture. Thus it is subjected to severe strains and stresses during all those daily activities that involve forward flextion of the body, for example, stooping or bending in the house and garden, or in many sporting activities. A normal healthy spinal column, after prolonged flexion of the back in such pursuits, may find difficulty in regaining the erect posture and the degree of stiffness will depend on the length of time that person has been in the stooped position. A moderately severe injury to the spinal column, for example a whiplash injury, may also cause a strain or sprain in the affected segment of spinal column, with stretching of a spinal joint and partial rupture of some of its ligaments, including quite often the ligamenta flava. Some patients suffering very acute pain in their mid-lumbar area, seem apparently locked in forward flexion in this lumbar segment of the spinal column. The patient is doubled over like a half-shut knife. The posterior back muscles particularly the erector spinati at the site of the spinal strain are in acute spasm. Putting the muscles in the affected region into spasm in order to reduce movement to a minimum, is Nature's way of relieving pain and preventing further damage to the affected muscles.

The condition is often confused with a slipped disc lesion or the locking of a facet joint. Diagnosis under x-ray is unhelpful, for it is always negative. Careful examination of the patient will show no past history of a back complaint or secondary features, such as sciatica or lumbago. These patients present a typical picture of the over-stretching of the elastic-like ligamenta flava which have temporarily lost their elasticity and thus are unable to perform their normal function of regaining the erect posture.

Treatment

Treatment is given by injecting 2 cc of local anaesthesia into the muscles which are in spasm on both sides of the spinal column. The patients are advised to lie on their backs on a normal softish bed for seven days, not being allowed up during this time. A physiotherapist should carry out a light massage daily, particularly to the limbs, during this period. A simple analgesic such as paracetamol, one every four hours is given, and initially an injection of ¼ cc of morphia may be required. At the end of one week of immobilised bed-rest, the patient is allowed up, after being fitted with an elasticated surgical corset in an attempt to keep movement in the sprained spinal area to a minimum. The surgical support is discarded in two weeks. Thereafter the patient is put on a training programme to quickly regain the tone in the affected muscle groups and he should follow the same regime as that following a lumbar slipped disc lesion.

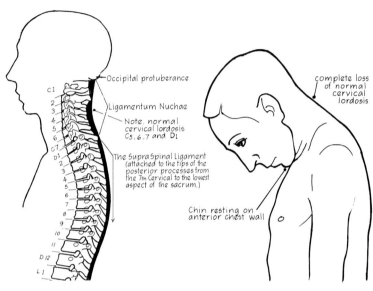

Diag. 74 Schematic lateral view of the normal cervical column showing the position of the ligamentum nuchae.

Diag. 75 A lateral view of the posture caused by the over-stretching of the ligamentum nuchae.

Labels in Diag. 74:
- Occipital protuberance
- C 1
- 2
- 3
- 4
- 5
- 6
- c 7
- D 1
- Ligamentum Nuchae
- Note. normal cervical lordosis C5, 6, 7 and D1
- The Supra Spinal Ligament (attached to the tips of the posterior processes from the 7th Cervical to the lowest aspect of the sacrum.)
- 2
- 3
- 4
- 5
- 6
- 7
- 8
- 9
- 10
- 11
- D 12
- L 1

Labels in Diag. 75:
- complete loss of normal cervical lordosis
- Chin resting on anterior chest wall

Diags. 74 and 75. The strain of the cervical ligament.

The Strain of the Cervical Ligaments

Overstraining and sprains of the cervical ligaments are quite a common occurrence, particularly as a result of the so-called whiplash injury. The posterior longitudinal ligament and the ligamentum nuchae are usually affected and quite often the disc complex also. This condition may also be a direct result of the daily occupation of the patient if that entails the head being held in forward flexion for long periods of time, e.g. surgeons, writers etc. The ligamentum nuchae is an elasticated fibrous ligament similar to the ligamenta flava except that it maintains and regains the head, (rather than the body), in the erect posture. Thus enforced forward flexion of the head for long periods can cause chronic strains in the ligament.

In the early stages of this condition, patients experience slight difficulty in raising the head but, in older age groups, the difficulty becomes more pronounced, for the condition is progressive. If the ligament becomes seriously overstretched, its elasticity may be permanently affected. The sufferer will then have great difficulty in raising his head. The chin is usually resting on his chest and one commonly sees the patient pushing his chin upwards and backwards in order to straighten his neck.

Treatment

After a careful clinical assessment of the case, and I have concluded that a disc lesion is not present, I prescribe a similar treatment as for the sprained ligamenta flava: complete rest including immobilisation of the cervical joints for about a week, followed by a prescribed training programme to tone up the muscles in the cervical area.

4. Spondylitis Deformans including "Poker Back"

As the two words "spondylitis deformans" have different meanings, I will define each separately and then explain how one condition progresses on to the other. "Spondylitis" means inflammation of the vertebra and "deformans", or "deformity" means distortion of any part or general disfigurement of the body, that is, the spinal vertebral body.

The condition begins with spondylitis, which is due to a non-specific inflammatory state of the spinal vertebrae which includes joint capsules, ligaments and intrinsic muscles and all periarticular

annular ligament   vertebral body

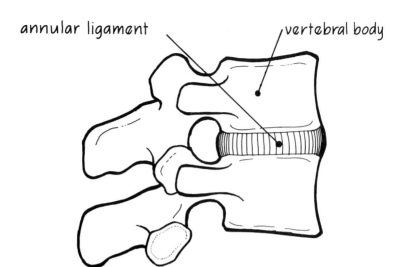

A. (above) lateral view of the normal disc complex.

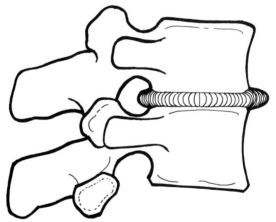

B. Note the marked flattening of the articular disc
complex, and the bulging of the annular ligament
in Spondylitis Deformans

Diag. 76. Spondylitis deformans.

tissues situated around the joints. To date no specific organism has been isolated from the affected joints or surrounding tissues. Thus the actual cause of this condition is still not completely known, although it has been the subject of much discussion and theorising. Within recent times, I have come to the conclusion that the condition is due to vertebral degeneration, regardless of age. The disease may start in childhood, but because early symptoms of muscle and joint pains are, as a rule, not severe enough to warrant investigation, the doctor may consider the clinical features to be nothing more than symptoms of growing pains, and in most cases, he will be right.

The condition may start with the clinical features of an acute infection but, in the majority of cases, it runs a more chronic course of infection of unknown origin, by the time it is clinically assessed. It is pointless to start relating all known organisms which perhaps could give rise to spondylitis as they do not qualify as a cause in most cases. Examination of blood has to date revealed very little, apart from a few cases with high uric acid, as in gout, or, as when the kidneys are infected, there may be an increase of the non-threshold substances, which normally filter through the kidneys. In my research, another important point has emerged. When one's health is impaired, a predisposing factor could well be exposure to cold, damp conditions. Injury also is a very definite factor as a cause of spondylitis. There are many other theories which, in my opinion, are nothing more than theory, at this particular stage of my research.

Following this acute phase, probably due to either spinal injury or exposure to cold and damp, a non-specific inflammation with acute pain in the affected area causes the muscles around the area to go into spasm, immobilising it in order to reduce pain. The acute phase, in time, would appear to burn itself out in many cases, but before this has occurred, treatment must be intense before the chronic state sets in.

In later stages, if the condition is left without treatment, deformity sets in, the capsules of joints become thickened, atrophied and then fibrosed: (in other words, the capsules start to waste and contract). The cartilages and articular surfaces may then be destroyed with decalcification of adjacent vertebral bodies. Fibrous adhesions may form between the bony surfaces, which may then ossify, or become bone. Changes occur in the annular ligaments and cartilage plates, and they may become fibrillated and eroded, exposing the bony surfaces of the vertebral bodies. Grooves form from the movements of the opposing surfaces and may cause crepitus (creaking). At the edges of the vertebrae, osteophytes, (bony outgrowths), may form and cause lipping which will reduce joint movement. True bony ankylosing (the joining of one bone to the other) may also occur in the spinal column. Muscle atrophy — wasting around the affected joints — always occurs, mostly due to disuse.

Deformity is always present due to contractures of capsules, ligaments and muscles, leading to bony distortion of the spinal column, with the resulting erosion of the disc or nucleus pulposus complex. This becomes flattened or distorted and may disappear.

SPONDYLITIS DEFORMANS can thus be defined as a deforming arthritis of the vertebral joints, causing the vertebral column to become bent and rigid. When the final stage of this disease sets in, it is called spondylosis. **Spondylosis simply means ankylosing,** which may be defined as an abnormal immobility and consolidation of a joint or joints. In the chronic state, there is a marked loss of movement in the affected spinal column with deformity which, at times, is gross.

Treatment

This should be undertaken immediately, i.e. as soon as the first symptoms of the acute phase presents itself. The patient should be put to bed, though not an orthopaedic bed. In some cases the condition may be the direct result of infection from a sceptic focus so a small blood sample, together with specimens of urine and faeces, should be sent to the laboratory in order to isolate possible causative organism or organisms and to assess uric acid content, in particular. If the blood sample proves positive, a massive dose of penicillin should be given (preferably by injection) providing, of course, that the patient is not allergic to this antibiotic. After the samples of urine and faeces have been taken, an enema should be given, followed by a strong laxative. At the same time, a strong diuretic should be given to clear the urinary tract and keep it functioning properly. As stated above, the disease could well be set up by faulty elimination of toxic products from urine or bowel matter. The patient is put onto a sugar free diet and kept at rest in bed for seven days. During this time he should receive gentle massage from the physiotherapist daily.

If the patient is seen for the first time in the sub-acute or early chronic phase of the disease, i.e. before deformity with gross loss of movement of the spinal column has set in, the investigation of blood, urine and faeces should be carried out, as in the acute case. The only difference is that the patient is not put to bed. In fact, he or she should gently go about his or her normal activities and I prescribe a training programme in order to keep all muscles gently active and thus, these in turn, will keep all joints, which they control, mobile. This mobility of joints stretches the muscles, ligaments and capsules which surround them and, by so doing, in time, prevents contractures and permanent immobility in the affected spinal joints and peri-articular tissues.

Even in the more chronic cases where there is very little movement in the affected joints, I prescribe a specific course of training and, at the same time, I physically move the involved joints, thus stretching their capsules and surrounding ligaments and muscles. The improvement following a course of this treatment can be, at times, quite dramatic.

This condition, which basically affects the spinal column, occurs most commonly in males and, in the majority of cases, there is history of heavy manual work or of injury to the spinal column. The cervical (neck) or upper thoracic regions are usually affected and these areas of the spinal column may become fixed by ankylosis (abnormal immobility and consolidation of a joint). The lumbar region may also be involved. Where the whole spinal column is implicated the condition is known as **"Poker Back" (Spondylitis Ankylopoetica).**

Normal Cervical Lordosis is lost.

Normal Dorsal Kyphosis is flattened.

Normal Lumbar Lordosis is lost.

Note that on forward flexion, the spinal column is completely rigid and flat. This is due to the contraction of the intrinsic muscles, ligaments, and capsules of the facet joints. In the final stages practically no movement is present in any part of the spinal column, hence the name 'Poker Back'.

Diag. 77. Spondylitis Ankylopoetica, 'Poker Back'.

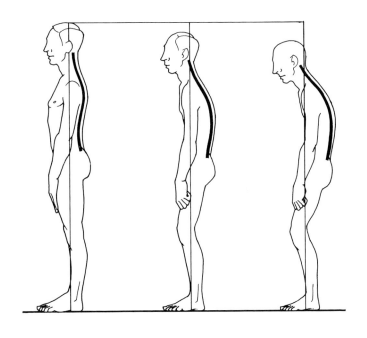

Normal Contour   The Ageing Man.   The Aged Man.

Diag. 78. The standing posture in the ageing process.

5. Spinal Deformities of the Aged

THE AGEING PROCESS

Figure I   **Normal Contour**

Note that the alignment of the vertebrae, one to the other, gives rise to the specific shape of the spinal column, but the column is maintained entirely by the surrounding muscles.

Figure II   **The Ageing Man**

NOTE: the slight forward flexion of the head
the slight rounding of the back
the flattening of the anterior chest wall
the slight forward flexion of the knee joints
the feet tend to flatten, with a loss of spring in walking.

In this posture, the patient's activities become grossly diminished. Thus stiffening of all joints follows with a varying degree of muscle wasting. The individual's balance may become seriously impaired.

Figure III   **The Aged Man**

NOTE: The Ageing processes, referred to in the notes of figure II above, become exaggerated, resulting in the contraction of joint capsules and muscle wasting; the stiffening and loss of movements in most of the joints and, of course, considerable loss of height, say 5″ or more. The patient's balance is impaired, giving him a tendency to fall forward. The erect posture is maintained by the compensatory action of bending the knees forward. The consequent reduction of mobility, in especially the joints of the lower limbs, may result in a shuffling gait.

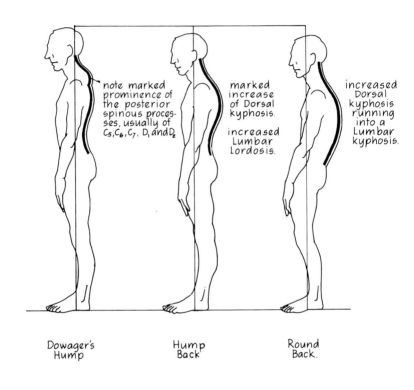

Diag. 79. Spinal deformities in the aged.

Spinal Deformities in the Aged

There are characteristics which we associate with the aged. When people reach the age of 70, or even younger, most accept the fact that the ageing process will leave them with a permanent stoop, or bowing of the back. Most people regard this as inevitable, for it can occur in the normal healthy ageing individual. Fortunately, this is not the case.

The normal contour of the spinal column is formed initially by the articulation of the vertebrae, one with the other, throughout the whole column. At the upper end the 1st cervical vertebra articulates with the condyles, or base of the skull, and at the lower aspect the 5th lumbar vertebra articulates with the upper surface of the sacrum. The specific alignment of the column is thus formed by the articulation of these joints, but this normal contour is entirely controlled and maintained by the muscles that surround and control the column. Thus any weakness of this musculature may cause deformities to arise in the column.

As one gets older, one tends to become less and less active. This leads to a disuse atrophy of the muscular system which, in turn, diminishes joint movement, with the inevitable contraction of the joint capsules. Thus varying degrees of joint stiffness will ensue, often causing pain. The pain will again limit movement and the condition will accelerate, varying naturally from person to person. The patient will gradually become thinner with a marked loss of tone in the muscle groups, which normally move the affected joint or joints.

The diminished joint movement and contraction of the joint capsules cause deformities to arise affecting the whole length of the spinal column.

1. **Cervical area.** Commonly, the head is held slightly forward and its weight gradually flattens the normal cervical lordosis. This may extend as far as the upper Dorsal vertebrae and involve D.2 and D.3. It leads to the prominence of the posterior spinous processes, usually of C.5, C.6, C.7, D.1 and D.2. This condition is known as "Dowager's Hump" and usually, particularly in females, a pad of fat is superimposed over these processes. Usually associated with this condition, a rounding of the shoulders occurs, due to lack of tone in the posterior muscles of the shoulder joints.

2. **Dorsal area.** In the dorsal region of the spinal column, the normal kyphosis increases and if this becomes gross we refer to it as "Dorsal Round Back", or "Hump Back".

3. **Lumbar area.** If the muscle wasting process continues into the lumbar region, the normal lumbar lordosis decreases, giving rise to a marked reduction of the hollow in the lower back. In many cases, there is a complete reversal of the lumbar lordosis, producing a lumbar kyphosis. This deformity will join up with the dorsal kyphosis in the condition known as complete "Round Back".

4. **Lower limbs.** The older person tends to bend forwards and may often fall forwards if his balance is seriously impaired. He may unconsciously seek to restore his balance by a slight forward flexion of the knee joints. This affects the gait of that person, because walking with the knee joints in forward flexion quite quickly weakens the musculature of the lower limbs, and, in many older age groups, this results in a shuffling gait. In these cases, extra stress is exerted on to the feet, which, in turn, leads to the flattening of the longitudinal arches, with added instability and diminished walking ability.

Usually there is a thinning of the annular ligaments between opposing vertebral bodies, which as a rule, leads to a marked loss of height from 3 to 7 inches.

These deformities obviously vary from individual to individual and are usually slower to develop in the healthy ageing person. They are nevertheless accepted by almost everyone as part of the normal process of growing old. I believe that such deformites can be prevented by a twice daily routine of exercises. The specific training programmes I prescribe, are devised to prevent and/or correct the exaggerated forward flexion of the cervical (neck), dorsal (chest) and, at times, lumbar (lower back) regions of the spinal column. All these exercises act specifically on all muscles in the posterior aspect of the whole spinal column which have lost their tone and power. Thus they tone in turn, all the muscles of the posterior cervical area, the posterior supra-scapular muscles, the posterior muscles of the shoulder girdle, all the muscles of the posterior dorsal area and finally all the muscles of the posterior lumbar region. I have devised further exercises to tone up the muscles and joints of the lower limbs.

If a deformity has already begun to develop, 'surgical' manipulation may well be required to correct the abormal curvature of the spinal column. Thereafter, the patient must exercise rigorously and with perseverance, to tone up the muscles, that, most probably, are atrophied from disuse, in order to gain full mobility of all the joints concerned.

162

Methods of Slowing Down the Deformities of the Aged

1. **Methods to prevent and correct the deformity in the neck or cervical area, commonly called "Dowager's Hump"**

In most cases, this condition starts to develop over the age of 40. The cause of it, usually, apart from trauma, or injury, is postural and often has a direct bearing on the patient's occupation, during which the head is bent forward for prolonged periods. In point of fact, most everyday actions of the head involve forward flextion, for example eating, writing, stooping and most sports. Even in sleep, our heads usually rest bending forwards. Very rarely, do we bend our heads backwards — perhaps occasionally to look at the sky etc. Not more than possibly 5-10 seconds in 24 hours are given to backward extension of the head.

In the lower cervical spinal column, there is a slight to moderate normal forward angulation (cervical lordosis) at C.5/6/7/D.1 and the weight of the head is constantly bearing down on this angulation. It is exactly at this level that the cervical or Dowager's hump develops.

This condition has quite a distinct family background. It is fairly common for the patient to inform me that her mother, grandmother or an older sister has a similar deformity. I have examined older members of the family and some did have the deformity but, in many cases, had no symptoms. It was quite interesting to note that the members of the family in question appeared to have adopted the same postural habit.

Generally speaking, however, in patients suffering from this condition, the posterior neck muscles are liable to become overstretched and the anterior aspects of the annular ligaments become flattened. The facet joints may be pulled apart, with the overstretching of their intrinsic ligaments and muscles.

However, some patients with this condition are referred to me by their doctor because of their neurological symptoms, for example brachial neuritis or post occipital neuritis with headaches, which, at times, have a migraine-like syndrome. In these cases, x-ray usually reveals a narrowing of the space between C.6/7 and, at times, of the space between C.5/6 or C.7/D.1, indicating a disc lesion. At this level, the lateral x-ray will usually show a slight to moderate kyphosis, early spondylosis and early slight to moderate osteoarthritis.

In these cases, the disc is detached non-surgically, as described in Chapter VI, and 'surgical' manipulation given to stretch the affected intrinsic muscles and ligaments. A training programme of exercises is prescribed, and these are again described in Chapter VI. Such treatment also corrects the effects of early arthritis by rubbing one rough surface of the joints against the other until the surfaces become smooth and polished (eburnated) and thus move more easily and painlessly.

Where there is no disc lesion, and the condition is gross, 'surgical' manipulation may still be necessary. Thereafter, and in cases where the condition is still slight, I recommend the training programme prescribed for patients with cervical disc lesions referred to above and described in Chapter VI and Appendix IIC.

2. Methods to prevent and correct the deformity in the Dorsal area.

As the "Round Back" condition progresses, it becomes increasingly difficult to take deep breaths. These are essential for the wellbeing of an active patient and a good supply of oxygen is necessary for muscle building. After 'surgical' manipulation, if required, I advise a patient, suffering from a "Round Back", to carry out the training programme prescribed for patients suffering from dorsal disc lesions that I describe in Chapter VII and Appendix IID. They should be done twice daily, the patient being sure to take deep breaths throughout the exercises.

3. Methods to prevent and correct the deformity in the lumbar area.

If the normal lumbar lordosis has increased considerably, 'surgical' manipulation may be necessary. During this course of treatment, and afterwards, the patient should perform the set of exercises prescribed for patients suffering from a disc lesion in the lumbar region. These are described in Chapter V and Appendix IIA.

Regular exercise will undoubtedly retard the ageing process, for it tones the muscles and keeps the joints mobile and relatively pain free. The spinal column relies on the tone of the associated muscles to support it in its normal alignment. Any weakness in the musculature supporting the column will result in deformity. Thus it is beneficial to exercise systematically, following the training programme I have designed specifically to tone these muscles, exercising in turn each set of muscles which supports the three areas of the spinal column. It is recommended that everyone should acquire the habit of twice daily exercise as part of the their normal day, so that it becomes as routine as washing or the cleaning of teeth.

164

Conclusion

In conclusion, I should like to summarise my whole thesis about the condition of the slipped disc, and I make no apologies for repetition. Every day in my surgery I am asked the same questions, all of which betray a fundamental misunderstanding of this problem.

The vertebral bodies of the spinal column are separated and cushioned by a ring of fibro-cartilage called the annular ligament. Through constant wear and tear or subjection to excessive strain during an accident, a cut or tear may occur in the ligament, and the jelly-like disc contained within it, will then protrude through this tear. If this disc strikes a nerve root, it causes the excessive pain, that is the crippling symptom of the slipped disc condition.

My treatment consists of detaching this protruding disc and this enables the tear in the ligament to heal. Because of my knowledge of the intricate mechanism of the spinal column, I am able, in the course of my treatment, to break off the protruding portion of the disc with my thumb under a local anaesthetic. The detached pieces of disc will now atrophy and usually pass out of the system as waste products. The disc when completely eradicated can, therefore, never again 'slip out', and cause any further discomfort. The vertebrae do not come closer together as a result of this treatment, for the disc only is detached, leaving the annular ligament to fulfil its normal function as a buffer or cushion between the vertebral bodies. This ligament is so strong, being made up of fibro-cartilaginous rings, that the removal of the disc does not weaken it.

Some deformities of the spinal column may have occurred if the 'slipped disc' has been left untreated for a time. Initially, I treat this condition by 'surgical' manipulation to correct the deformity, and I also prescribe a training programme to strengthen those muscles that will keep the spinal column in the normal alignment, into which I have placed it by manipulation.

I recommend the practice of further exercises, because the correct position of the spinal column is largely maintained by strong muscular support. This will, therefore, prevent abnormal strain on the other parts of the column.

Chapters IV, V, VI and VII have described the treatment I have been practising in my surgery over the last thirty years. Quite literally, several thousands of patients have come for consultation and treatment and the very high success rate achieved, has convinced me of the value of my treatment.

My own personal satisfaction has not, however been in the justification of the theory for its own sake. The only true satisfaction that a doctor can achieve is the knowledge that, through his treatment, he has cured a painful condition, or at the very least, alleviated suffering. My patients have given me ample proof that I have been able to do so. At the same time, my life has been enriched by the opportunity to meet so many interesting people from all walks of life, who have visited me in my surgery and, in many cases, extended my experience of life through their own enthusiastic involvement in full and varied careers.

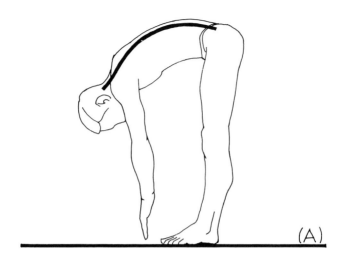

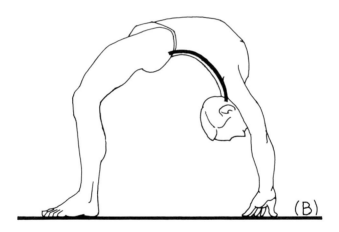

Note the diminished forward flexion and the greater backward extension of the lumbar spinal column. This normal anatomical fact is used to advantage in the modern method of high-jumping.

Diag. 80. (A) Forward flexion and (B) backward extension, of the spinal column.

APPENDIX I

Further Anatomical Details of the Spinal Column

Movements of the Spinal Column

THE SPINAL column is capable of a wide range of movement, flexion, extension, circumduction and rotation. Adjacent vertebrae articulate with each other by their bodies, through the intervention of the intervertebral disc complex and through their articular processes, i.e. facets. The variety of movements is influenced by the shape and direction of the articular surfaces.

In flexion and forward movement, the anterior longitudinal ligament is relaxed and the annular ligament is compressed in front, whilst the posterior longitudinal, the ligamenta flava, and the inter and supraspinal ligaments are stretched, as well as the posterior fibres of the annular ligament. The interspaces between the laminae are widened and the inferior articular processes (or facets) glide upwards upon the superior articular processes (or facets) of the subjacent vertebrae.

Extension is the most extensive of all the movements of the vertebral column and compared with flexion an exactly opposite disposition of the parts takes place. This movement is limited by the anterior longitudinal ligament and by the approximation of the spinous processes, particularly the posterior ones. It is quite free in the cervical region and most free in the lumbar area.

The modern method of the high jump in athletics is developed from the realisation that greater movement can be obtained by making use of the backward extension of the lumbar column, than from jumping in a forward flexion position. Thus in the high jump, the athlete jumps with the bar to his back, leading with his head, thus taking full advantage of the greater hollow of the mid-lumbar regions

In lateral movements, the sides of the annular ligaments are compressed, the extent of the motion being limited by the resistance offered by the surrounding ligaments. This movement may take place in any part of the column, but is most free in the cervical and lumbar regions.

Circumduction is very limited and is merely a succession of the preceding movements. **Rotation** is produced by the twisting of the intervertebral complex. This, although only slight between any two vertebrae, allows of a considerable extent of movement when it takes place in the whole length of the column, the front upper part of the column being turned to one side or the other. This movement occurs to a slight extent in the cervical region, is more free in the upper part of the thoracic region and is absent in the lumbar region.

All these movements are influenced in their extent and variety by the shape and direction of the articular surfaces and as these can vary quite considerably from one individual to another with normal healthy spinal columns, so also does the extent of movements vary among normal healthy human beings.

In the Cervical region the upward inclination of these facets allows free flexion and extension. Extension can be carried further than flexion (a feature many leading anatomical text books would not confirm). At the upper end of the region it is checked by the locking of the posterior edges of the superior atlantal facets in the condyloid fossae of the occipital bone. At the lower end it is limited by a mechanism whereby the inferior articular processes of the seventh cervical vertebra slip into grooves behind and below the superior articular processes of the first thoracic. Flexion is arrested just beyond the point where the cervical convexity is straightened. The movement is checked by the opposition of the projecting lower lips of the bodies of the vertebrae. Lateral flexion and rotation are free in the cervical region. They are, however, always combined. The upwards and medial inclinations of the superior (facet) articular surfaces impart a rotary movement during lateral flexion whilst pure rotation is prevented by the slight medial shape of these surfaces.

In the thoracic region, notably in its upper part, all the movements are limited in order to reduce interference with respiration to a minimum. The almost complete absence of an upward inclination of the superior articular surfaces prohibits any marked flexion, while extension is checked by the contact of the posterior spinous processes with one another. Rotation is free in the thoracic region. The superior articular surfaces are segments of a cylinder whose axis is in the mid-ventral line of the vertebral bodies. The direction of the articular facets would allow free lateral flexion, but this movement is considerably limited in the upper part of the region by the resistance of the ribs and sternum.

In the lumbar region flexion and extension are free. The inferior articular facets are not in close opposition with the superior facets of the adjacent vertebrae and, on this account a considerable amount of lateral flexion is permitted. For the same reason a slight amount of rotation can be carried out, but this is soon checked by the interlocking of the facet joints. Overall the movement in backward flexion is greater than that obtained in forward flexion and vertical extension.

The Muscles used in Spinal Movement

The principal muscles which produce **flexion** are the sterno cleido mastoideus, longus capitis and longus colli, the scaleni, the abdominal muscles and the psoas major. **Extension** is produced by the intrinsic muscles of the back, assisted in the neck by the splenius, semispinales dorsi and cervices and the multifidus. **Lateral rotation** is produced by the intrinsic muscles of the back: by the splenius, the scaleni, the quadratus lumborum and the psoas major, the muscles of one side only, acting. **Rotation** is produced by the action of the following muscles, again acting on one side only. These are the sterno cleido mastoideus, the longus capitus, the scaleni, the multifidus, the semispinalis capitis and the abdominal muscles.

The Ligaments of the Spinal Column

The supporting structures of the spinal joints may be divided into two groups; the muscles which form the active group and the ligaments which are largely passive. The opposing surfaces of the spinal vertebrae are held together by the following ligaments.

1. The Intervertebral Annular Ligament

This is situated between the adjacent surfaces of the bodies of the vertebrae and constitute the chief bond of union between them. Through its elasticity, it permits movement or compression of the spinal column to a moderate degree. It acts as a spring, to allow movement but also acts as a cushion or buffer, enabling the column to withstand jolts or jars caused by fierce movement or sudden actions. It encloses the soft nucleus pulposus or disc and only, when damaged, allows this to protrude, giving rise to a slipped disc lesion. Its detailed anatomy has been given earlier in Chapter I, page 39.

2. The Posterior Longitudinal Ligament is situated within the spinal canal and extends over the posterior surfaces of the bodies of the

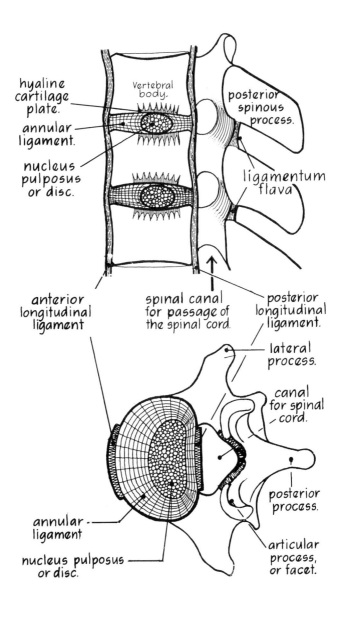

Diag. 81. Schematic views of the spinal column, showing ligamentum flava, and posterior and anterior longitudinal ligaments.

174

vertebrae and the annular ligaments. It is broader above than below and consists of glistening fibres which extend from the axis (which is the second cervical vertebra) to the first coccygeal vertebra — its sacral part, however, being very narrow and delicate. The fibres are firmly attached to the annular ligament and the margins of the vertebral bodies, but they are separated from the centres of the bodies by the transverse venous communication between the anterior intraspinal veins. In the cervical region, the ligament is of almost uniform breadth, being expanded over the vertebral bodies as well as over the annular ligament. In the thoracic and lumbar regions, however, it is narrow opposite the vertebral bodies and broad opposite the annular ligaments. The arrangement of its fibres is similar to the arrangement of those of the anterior longitudinal ligament. The posterior longitudinal ligament is serially continuous superiorly with the posterior occipito-axial ligament.

The clinical importance of the posterior common or longitudinal ligament has a specific bearing on the slipped disc lesion, because of its firm anatomical attachment to the annular ligament which, in turn, connects with, and surrounds, the nucleus pulposus or disc. Thus overstretching of the posterior longitudinal ligament, by continued forward flexion (as in toe touching) of the spinal column, causes the annular ligament to be pulled backwards leading to gradual thinning of the annular ligament. In time, perhaps following a minor injury to the spinal column, the disc bursts through the remaining fibres of the thinned annular ligament leading to a slipped disc lesion but the presence of the posterior longitudinal ligament prevents damage by the slipped disc to the spinal cord. A disc, therefore, usually prolapses postero-laterally at the weakest and unprotected point of the thinned annular ligament and, very often, strikes a nerve root in this position.

3. **The Anterior Longitudinal Ligament**

This is a dense band of white glistening fibres, which extends over the anterior surfaces of the bodies of the vertebrae and annular ligaments. It extends from the axis to the first segment of the sacrum and its fibres are disposed longitudinally. The most superficial fibres extend from a given vertebra to the fifth below it. The deepest fibres pass from a given vertebra to the one immediately below it. The fibres are firmly attached to the annular ligament and margins of the vertebral bodies, but very loosely to the centres of the bodies on account of the presence of the blood vessels. The anterior longitudinal ligament is broadest in the lumbar region and thickest in the thoracic

175

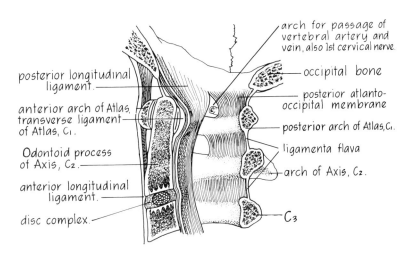

posterior longitudinal ligament.

anterior arch of Atlas, transverse ligament of Atlas, C₁.

Odontoid process of Axis, C₂.

anterior longitudinal ligament.

disc complex.

arch for passage of vertebral artery and vein, also 1st cervical nerve.

occipital bone

posterior atlanto-occipital membrane

posterior arch of Atlas, C₁.

ligamenta flava

arch of Axis, C₂.

C₃

A. (above) Schematic lateral section of the occipital bone and the first three cervical vertebrae.

B. (below) Schematic posterior veiw of the occipital bone and the first three cervical vertebrae.

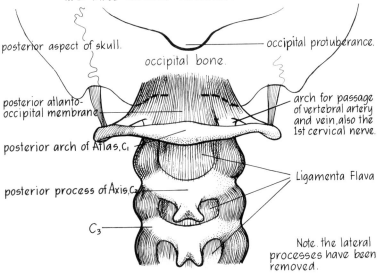

posterior aspect of skull.

occipital protuberance.

occipital bone.

posterior atlanto-occipital membrane

arch for passage of vertebral artery and vein, also the 1st cervical nerve.

posterior arch of Atlas, C₁

posterior process of Axis, C₂

Ligamenta Flava

C₃

Note. the lateral processes have been removed.

Diag. 82. Upper cervical ligaments.

176

region. It is thicker opposite the centres of the bodies than elsewhere and in these situations it fills up the cavities and so renders the column less undulating than it otherwise would be. Over the lateral surfaces of the bodies, a few scattered fibres are present, which pass from one vertebra to that below. In the sacral region, the anterior longitudinal ligament is lost in the periosteum of the bone, but it appears lower down as the anterior sacro-coccygeal ligament. The anterior longitudinal ligament is serially continuous superiorly with the anterior atlanto-axial ligament.

4. The Ligamenta Flava

The importance of these elasticised ligaments cannot be too strongly stressed. They form a structure that, in the past, has been taken for granted and thus very little has been written about it, apart from a description of its presence, in anatomical text books. It is a very important structure clinically, particularly if one considers its function physically. It is made up of sections of elastic tissue attached to, and extending between, the ventral adjacent portions of the arches of the vertebrae. It connects the laminae of the adjacent vertebrae from the atlas to the first segment of the sacrum and is best seen from the interior of the vertebral canal. It extends from the articular capsules to the point where the laminae fuse to form the spinous process. Here their posterior margins come into contact and are, to a certain extent, united, small intervals being left for the passage of vessels. The ligamenta flava consists of yellow elastic tissues, the fibres of which are almost perpendicular in direction. They are attached to the anterior surface of the laminae above — some distance from its inferior margin — and to the posterior surface and upper margin of the laminae below. In the cervical region, the ligaments are thin, but broad and long. They are thicker in the thoracic region and thickest in the lumbar region. Its essential function is that it assists in maintaining or regaining the erect posture. It serves also to close in the spaces between the arches of the vertebrae.

Its most important characteristic is its strong elasticated fibres which assist, to a far greater extent than was previously ascribed to this ligament, in maintaining or regaining the erect posture. It is subjected to severe stresses and strains during one's daily normal activities; for example, in every act which causes one to stoop down to pick something from the ground; to put on socks or stockings; to tie one's shoe laces — in fact every type of physical movement which demands forward flexion of the spinal column and this, of course, includes most of all forms of sport and gardening.

177

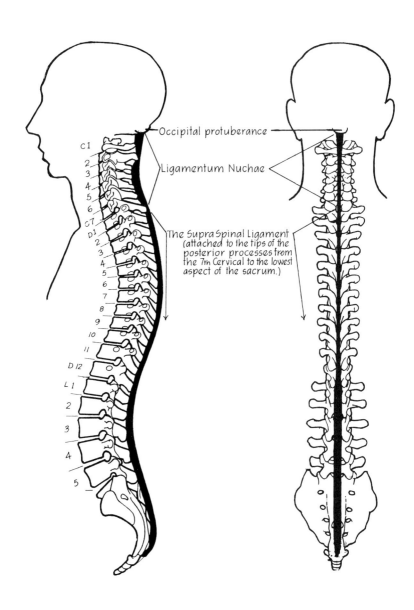

Diag. 83. Schematic views of the ligamentum nuchae and the supraspinal ligament.

178

With a perfectly normal healthy spinal column after prolonged forward flexion of the back, an individual often has some difficulty in regaining the erect posture. The degree of stiffness depends on the length of time that person has been in the stooped position. Quite often patients are brought to me suffering very acute pain in their mid-lumbar area with their spinal column apparently locked in forward flexion in the lumbar segment of the spinal column. Careful examination of the patient reveals no history of a back complaint nor shows any secondary features such as sciatica or lumbago from a previous disc lesion. These patients present a typical picture of overstretching of the elastic like ligamenta flava. The structure has temporarily lost its elasticity and thus is unable to perform its normal function of regaining the erect posture. The treatment for such a condition is given in Chapter IX, page 150.

5. The Supraspinal Ligament

This is a strong fibrous cord which connects together all the posterior spinous processes from the seventh cervical vertebra to the sacrum, the points of attachments being at the tips of the spinous processes. Fibro cartilage is developed in the ligament. It is thicker and broader in the lumbar region than in the thoracic region and is intimately blended in both situations with the neighbouring fascia. The most superficial fibres of this ligament extend over three or four vertebrae. Those more deeply seated pass between two or three vertebrae, while the deepest connect the spinous processes of the neighbouring vertebrae. Between the spinous processes the ligament is continuous with the interspinal ligaments. Between the spinous process of the seventh cervical vertebra and the external occipital protruberance, its place is taken by the ligamentum nuchae.

6. The Ligamentum Nuchae

This is a fibrous membrane which, in the neck, represents the supraspinal ligaments of the lower vertebrae. It extends from the external protruberance and median nuchan line of the occipital bone to the spinous process of the seventh cervical vertebra. From its anterior border, a fibrous lamina is given off, which is attached to the posterior tubercle of the atlas and to the spinous processes of the cervical vertebrae and forms a septum between the muscles on either side of the neck. In man it is the representative of an important elastic ligament, which in some lower animals, serves to sustain the weight of the head.

Overstraining and sprains of this, the cervical ligament, is quite common and patients may have slight difficulty in raising the head or, in chronic cases, the chin will rest on the chest and the patient has to push his chin upwards and backwards, to straighten his neck. Clinically, this is similar to the overstretching of the ligamenta flava and the treatment is similar, and described in Chapter IX, page 153.

7. Ligamenta Denticulata

These are twenty toothed processes extending from the pia mater to the dura mater pushing the arachnoid before them. They leave the pia midway between the anterior and posterior nerve roots and serve to suspend the cord in the mid line. The lowest ligamentum denticulatum is forked and the posterior root of the first lumbar nerve lies on the outer prong of the fork. In the lower region of the cord, it is the surgeon's guide to the first lumbar nerve and gives him a nerve root of a known number from which he can determine the position of the nerve roots.

8. The Interspinal Ligaments

These are thin and membraneous and connect adjoining spinous processes, extending from the root to the apex of each process. They meet the ligamenta flava in front and the supraspinal ligament behind. They are narrow and elongated in the thoracic region; broader, thicker and quadrilateral in form in the lumber region, and only slightly developed in the neck.

9. The Intertransverse Ligaments

These are interposed between the transverse processes. In the cervical region they consist of a few irregularly scattered fibres. In the thoracic region, they are rounded cords, intimately connected with the deep muscles of the back. In the lumbar region, they are thin and membraneous.

These ligaments are concerned, together with the facet joints, the muscles and ligaments, with the varied movements of the spinal column.

APPENDIX II

IN THIS appendix I have summarised the advice I give to those patients suffering from A) lumbago B) sciatica C) a cervical disc lesion and D) a dorsal disc lesion.

These summaries follow a similar pattern: first explaining the condition and my method of treatment, then secondly, describing the routine training programme suitable for that patient and finally, giving advice on how to alleviate the residual symptoms that may persist for a while after the treatment.

They were conceived originally as "hand-outs", intended to be given separately to each patient, (if desired), to provide a brief, but comprehensive, explanation of his particular condition. Thus they were written to be self sufficient, without reference to each other or to the main text. Repetition is therefore inevitable.

Advice to Patients Suffering from a Slipped Disc Lesion in the Lumbar Region, Causing Lumbago

What is a slipped disc?

A SLIPPED disc condition arises when injury, or a summation of minor injuries, causes a tear in the annular ligament that surrounds the disc. This allows the disc to prolapse through the tear and if that disc strikes a nerve root, intense pain will ensue. Once a disc has struck a nerve root, pain will continue in the hypersensitive nerve, leading to a spasm of all muscles supplied by that nerve. This gives rise in the lumbar region to an acute lumbago, amounting to a marked spasm of the lumbar muscles which are affected. At the same time, these muscles which are in spasm, will pull the spinal column towards them, giving rise to a scoliosis i.e. a lateral twisting of the spinal column to the affected side.

Treatment

The pain and other symptoms will persist as long as the disc mechanically presses on the nerve root. This is the prime cause of the symptoms, and I make it my policy to treat the cause and not the symptoms, for they will disappear in their own time, once the treatment has been achieved. In order to effect a permanent cure, the disc must be detached from its source of nutrient and allowed to atrophy. This I do manually under local anaesthesia and, at the first treatment, detach all the disc that is protruding through the tear in the annular ligament. During successive treatments, three or four in all, more disc will protrude during the gentle activity of the patient, and be detached similarly until it is all cleared away, usually within a fortnight.

Concurrently, during the same appointments, manipulation is carried out to correct the scoliosis formed by muscle spasm. Audible clicks may be heard during this process but this is not the disc being 'put back', as is often thought, but the clicking of one bony facet over another. The disc is, in fact, jelly-like and cannot either be 'put back' or cause any clicking sound.

The Training Programme

Muscles that are in spasm, caused by the mechanical pressure of the disc on the nerve root supplying those muscles, are not in good tone. Thus I prescribe a training programme to regain tone in the affected muscles. The prescribed exercises must not be neglected, for the muscles must eventually be toned up to support the back in its normal alignment. The daily performance of the exercises contained in this programme calls for some patience and perseverance if the condition is longstanding. It must be remembered also that muscles will quickly lose their tone if they are not kept active and that oxygen is essential for muscle building, so deep breaths must always be taken when performing the exercises.

The Training Programme for Lumbar Disc Lesions

Exercise I (Lumbar)

Muscle Toning Traction

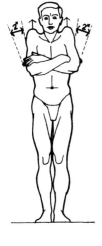

1. Stand erect with feet together.
2. Expand chest — this increases lumbar curve.
3. Fold arms across chest.
4. Raise points of shoulders to ears.
5. In this posture move the chest for 2″ from side to side, 25 times each way, bending through waist.
6. Take a deep breath with each movement. The shoulders should remain fixed in this position. It is the chest which moves from side to side and, at the same time, it is being pulled upwards all the time.

Diag. 84.

184

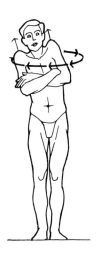

Exercise II (Lumbar)

Spinal Rotation

1. Adopt the same posture as in Exercise I.
2. Rotate the chest through the waistline round and round for no more than 2″ from the vertical — first 20 times in one direction and then 20 times in the other direction.

Diag. 85

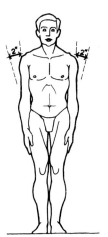

Exercise III (Lumbar)

Pendulum Movement of the Trunk

1. Stand in the erect posture with the arms kept at the side of the body.
2. Keep the chest expanded which increases the lumbar lordosis.
3. Flex the chest laterally 25 times from side to side, 2″ in either direction at speed. Bend at waist only. Do not move legs. The shoulders are held fixed and should only move with the chest.

Diag. 86.

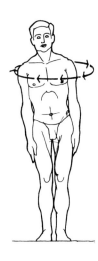

Exercise IV (Lumbar)

Rotation of the Trunk through the Waistline

1. Stand in the erect posture, as in exercise III.

2. Rotate the chest, bending at waistline only, not more than 2″, 25 times in one direction and 25 times in the other.

3. Arms kept close to body.

4. Shoulders should not be raised, but move with the chest.

Diag. 87.

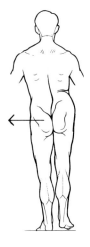

Exercise V (Lumbar)

Pelvic Jerk

This should be done if scoliosis is present, for it helps to pull the affected muscles out of spasm and straightens the spinal column. In the erect posture, jerk the pelvis from the affected side straight across to the unaffected side.

1. Jerk the pelvis from the affected side straight across to the unaffected side, i.e. from right to left, 20 jerks four times per day.

Diag. 88.

186

Exercise I was devised to take the place of traction and is designed specifically to produce a slight extension of the spinal column through the waistline. Exercise II produces a rotation of the column and has the effect of compressing the column, thus extruding further portions of disc through the tear in the annular ligament.

If the patients follow this training programme they are helping me to help themselves get fit and they are usually cured within 10-14 days. However, in some cases symptoms can be slow to clear depending, possibly on the length of time the patient has been suffering. Also in the older age groups, patients' symptoms are somewhat slower to clear up. In 2-3% of cases, pain may persist or recur over many months. It helps if the patient understands why, in these cases, pain still persists. When a slipped disc has been striking a nerve root for a considerable time, the nerve will have become very, very sensititve, and will remain so for a time after the striking has been discontinued. In a similar way, the pain from a blow on the chin lasts much longer than the actual blow and the injured area remains sensitive for an appreciable time.

The following advice is given as a guideline to the patient to help him to cope with these persisting symptoms, explaining which activities will cause distress and those that will alleviate discomfort. It is very important to avoid any state which will aggravate the condition.

Activities which Aggravate Lumbago

1. **Lying on a 'hard board' bed.** The human body has many prominences which become painful when they press on a hard surface. If one lies on one's side the point of the shoulder and the side of the hip joint become sore. When one lies on one's back the posterior aspect of the shoulder blades and the fixed sacrum below become painful. Also if these prominences are not cushioned, the remainder of the spinal column falls towards the hard surface, thus aggravating the condition.

2. **Sitting on a hard seat.** The weight of the trunk presses downwards onto the painful muscles and in cases where the sciatic nerve is affected, the nerve is compressed onto the bony sciatic notch of the pelvis.

3. **Crossing legs.** This pulls on the painful spastic muscle area, thus aggravating the condition.

187

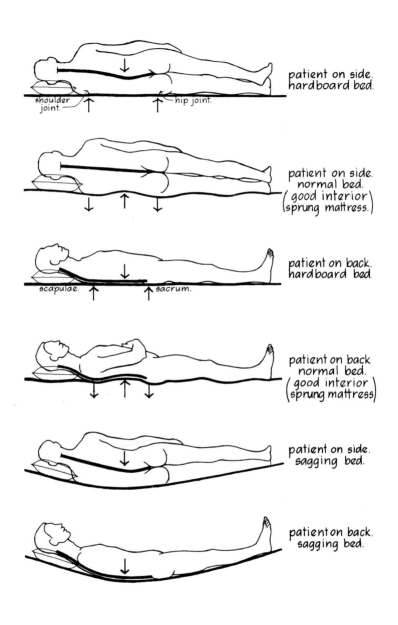

Diag. 89. Sleeping postures.

188

4. **Standing in the erect posture for any length of time.** The weight of the trunk presses down on the hypersensitive nerve root.

5. Taking long strides when walking. This pulls on the sensitive affected nerve, which, in turn, intensifies the lumbago.

6. **Toe Touching.** This stretches the muscles which are in spasm, thus increasing the lumbar pain.

7. **Lifting Heavy Loads.** Lifting heavy loads should be avoided, as far as possible, for two weeks. Patients when lifting anything, even the smallest item, should bend the knees, keeping the back straight and take the full weight in the arms. Patients when tying shoe laces or putting on socks or tights should sit and draw the feet up towards them, rather than bend the back and reach down to floor level.

8. **Avoid Using the Vacuum Cleaner** for two weeks as the pulling backwards and forwards of the cleaner puts a considerable strain on the lumbar muscles, thus aggravating the condition.

9. **Diving** into a Swimming Pool. This may hyperextend the spinal column, thus aggravating the condition.

10. **Straight Leg Raising.** This pulls on the spastic muscle area, thus increasing the pain.

11. **Avoid all forms of Sport.** Squash, golf, tennis, hockey, football, rugby, badminton, all forms of athletics and sport which involve quick jerking movements must be discontinued until the condition has cleared up, usually at the end of two weeks.

12. **Driving a Car** should be avoided until the condition has cleared up. The stretching of the legs out to the pedal controls pulls on the hypersensitive spastic muscles of the lumbar area.

13. **Avoid,** as far as possible, **coughing or sneezing.** These cause a wave of pressure of the cerebro-spinal fluid that surrounds the brain and the whole of the spinal cord. This wave will strike the hypersensitive affected nerve root and cause sharp, sudden, intense pain.

14. **Surgical corsets and plaster casts** must not be used, as this use leads to a disuse atrophy in the lumbar muscles. Most patients find the use of these frustrating.

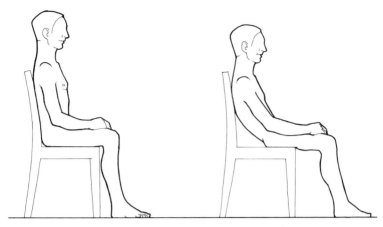

The correct way to sit on a chair. The lumbar curve is well supported.

Patients should never sit on the front edge of a chair as this causes the lumbar curve to be reversed.

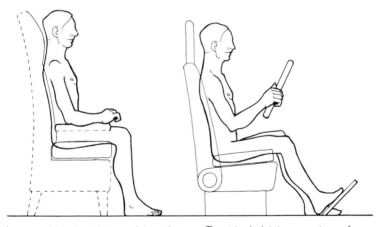

An easy chair should be upright with a well sprung back and seat. The patient should sit with his buttocks well back into the seat, (use additional cushions if necessary) and with his feet flat on the floor. The thighs should be at right-angles to the leg, with no pressure from the seat behind the knee joint.

The ideal driving posture for a back sufferer. Ensure the buttocks are well back, the driving wheel is close to the body, and the legs are always slightly flexed. Use a good, thick, well upholstered, latex-foam cushion on seat, and at the back, use additional cushions, if necessary.

Diag. 90. Seating postures recommended to alleviate lower lumbar pain.

Conditions which Alleviate Lumbago

1. **Sleep on a good interior sprung mattress.** This allows the affected area to mould into the mattress, whereas the 'hard board' bed causes pressure on the tender areas. It also ensures that the spinal contour is supported throughout its length.

2. **Sit on a soft seat, leaning slightly away from the painful area.** Sit right into the back of the chair to support the spinal column. Avoid a very low seat, even if it is soft, as you will have difficulty in regaining the erect posture.

3. **Sit on a thick rubber cushion in the bath.** Bend the knees slightly towards the chest, with slight lateral flexion of the body to the unaffected side.

4. **Stand with body weight onto the unaffected side** and slightly flex the body laterally to this side.

5. **Walk with short steps** to prevent pulling on affected muscles.

Advice to Patients Suffering from a Slipped Disc Lesion in the Lumbar Region Causing Sciatica

What is a Slipped Disc?

A SLIPPED disc condition arises when injury, or a summation of minor injuries, causes a tear in the annular ligament that surrounds the disc. This allows the disc to prolapse through the tear and if the disc strikes a nerve root, intense pain will ensue. If the disc strikes the sciatic nerve, then pain will be felt along the whole nerve tract, giving rise to pain in the buttocks on the affected side and extending down the leg, even as far as the toes. Sciatica is a symptom which can be very resistant to treatment. Pins and needles and some numbness may be felt as the pain diminishes after the initial treatments and this numbness is usually the last symptom to disappear, occasionally persisting some months after treatment.

It helps if the patient understands why, in some cases, pain still persists. When a slipped disc has been striking a nerve for a considerable time, the nerve will have become very, very sensitive. The pain from a blow on the chin lasts much longer than the actual blow and the injured area remains sensitive for an appreciable time. So, too, in some cases the sciatic nerve remains very sensitive and requires to be cushioned from external pressure or over-stretching.

The pressure of the disc on a hypersensitive nerve root will eventually lead to spasm of all muscles supplied by that nerve. These muscles in spasm will pull the spinal column towards them, leading to a scoliosis, or a lateral twisting of the spine towards the affected side.

193

Treatment

The root cause of all the symptoms is the mechanical pressure of the disc on the nerve root and thus this must be dealt with first. Once the cause of the pain has been eradicated, the symptoms will disappear in their own time. To effect a permanent cure, the disc must be detached from its source of nutrient and allowed to atrophy. The disc is detached manually, using my non-surgical technique, under local anaesthesia. At the first treatment I detach all the disc that is protruding through the tear in the annular ligament. During successive treatments, three or four in all, more disc will protrude during the gentle activity of the patient and be similarly detached until it is all cleared away, usually within a fortnight.

During the same appointments, manipulation is carried out to correct the scoliosis formed by muscle spasm. Audible clicks may be heard during this process, but this is not the disc being 'put back', as is often thought, but the clicking of one bony facet over another. The disc is, in fact, jelly-like and cannot either be 'put back' or cause any clicking sound.

The Training Programme

Muscles that are in spasm, caused by the mechanical pressure of the disc on the nerve root supplying those muscles, are not in good tone. Thus I prescribe a training programme to regain tone in the affected muscles. The prescribed exercises must not be neglected, for the muscles must eventually be strengthened to support the back in its normal alignment. The daily performance of the exercises contained in this programme calls for some patience and perseverance if the condition is to clear up, especially if scoliosis is present and the condition is long standing. It must be remembered also that muscles will quickly lose their tone if they are not kept active and that oxygen is essential for muscle building, so deep breaths must always be taken when performing the exercises.

The Training Programme for Lumbar Disc Lesions, Causing Sciatica

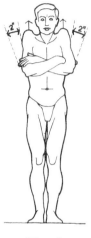

Diag. 91

Exercise I (Lumbar)

Muscle Toning Traction

1. Stand erect with feet together.

2. Expand chest — this increases lumbar curve.

3. Fold arms across chest.

4. Raise points of shoulders to ears.

5. In this posture, move the chest for 2″ from side to side 25 times each way, bending through waist.

6. Take a deep breath with each movement.
    The shoulders should remain fixed in this position. It is the chest which moves from side to side and, at the same time, it is being pulled upwards all the time.

195

Exercise II (Lumbar)

Spinal Rotation

1. Adopt the same posture as in Exercise I.

2. Rotate the chest through the waistline round and round for no more than 2″ from the vertical — first 20 times in one direction and then 20 times in the other direction.

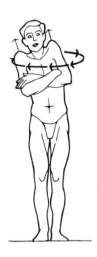

Diag. 92. (Exercise II)

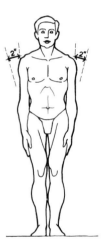

Diag. 93. (Exercise III)

Exercise III (Lumbar)

Pendulum Movement of the Trunk

1. Stand in the erect posture, with the arms kept at the side of the body.

2. Keep the chest expanded, which increases the lumbar lordosis.

3. Flex the chest laterally 25 times from side to side, 2″ in either direction at speed. Bend at waist only. Do not move legs. The shoulders are not raised and move with the chest.

Exercise IV (Lumbar)

Rotation of the Trunk through the Waistline

1. Stand in the erect posture as in Exercise III.
2. Rotate the chest, bending at waistline only, not more than 2″, 25 times in one direction and 25 times in the other.
3. Arms kept close to body.
4. Shoulders are not raised, but move with the chest.

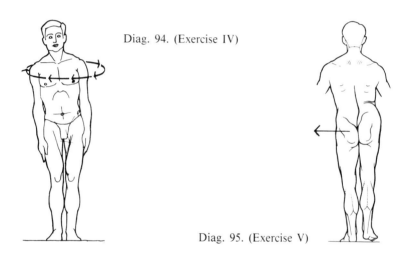

Diag. 94. (Exercise IV)

Diag. 95. (Exercise V)

Exercise V (Lumbar)

Pelvic Jerk

In cases of scoliosis where the column has been pulled to the right (see diagram)

1. Stand in the erect posture.
2. Jerk the pelvis from the affected side to the unaffected side, always coming back to the erect posture.
3. 20 jerks are carried out four times a day.

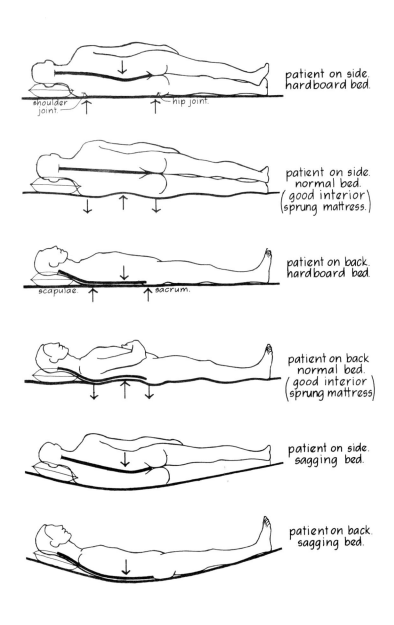

patient on side.
hardboard bed.

shoulder joint.   hip joint.

patient on side.
normal bed.
(good interior)
(sprung mattress.)

patient on back.
hardboard bed.

scapulae.   sacrum.

patient on back
normal bed.
(good interior)
(sprung mattress)

patient on side.
sagging bed.

patient on back.
sagging bed.

Diag. 96. Sleeping postures.

198

Exercise I was devised to take the place of traction and is designed specifically to produce a slight extension of the spinal column through the waistline. Exercise II produces a rotation of the column and has the effect of compressing it, thus extruding further portions of disc through the tear in the annular ligament.

If the patient follows this training programme he is helping himself to get fit and he is usually cured after 10-14 days. However, in 2-3% of cases and especially in the older age groups, pain or discomfort may persist and it is important to avoid any state which will aggravate the condition of the sensitive sciatic nerve. The following advice is given as a guideline to the patient to help him to cope with the persisting symptoms, explaining which activities will cause distress and those that will alleviate discomfort.

Activities which will Aggravate Sciatica

1. **Lying on a 'hard board' bed.** The human body has many bony prominences which become painful when they press on a hard surface. If one lies on one's side the point of the shoulder and the side of the hip joint become sore and when one lies on one's back the posterior aspect of the shoulder blades and the fixed sacrum below become painful. Also if these prominences are not cushioned the remainder of the spinal column falls onto the hard surface of the bed.

2. **Sitting on a hard seat.** The weight of the trunk presses straight down on to the acutely sensitive sciatic nerve. The nerve is compressed between the hard seat and the bony sciatic notch of the pelvis.

3. **Crossing Legs.** This pulls on the painful nerve.

4. **Standing in the erect posture for any length of time.** The weight of the trunk presses down on the hypersensitive nerve root.

5. **Taking long strides when walking.** This pulls on the sensitive affected nerve.

6. **Touching toes.** This stretches the muscles which are in spasm and stretches the very sensitive sciatic nerve.

7. **Lifting heavy Loads** should be avoided as far as possible for two weeks. Patients when lifting anything, even the smallest item, should bend the knees, keeping the back straight and take the full weight in the arms. Patients, when tying shoe laces or putting on socks or tights, should sit and draw the feet up towards them, rather than bend the back and reach down to floor level.

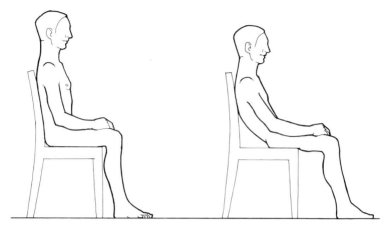

The correct way to sit on a chair. The lumbar curve is well supported.

Patients should never sit on the front edge of a chair as this causes the lumbar curve to be reversed.

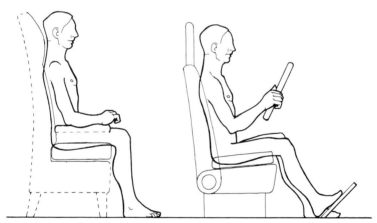

An easy chair should be upright with a well sprung back and seat. The patient should sit with his buttocks well back into the seat, (use additional cushions if necessary) and with his feet flat on the floor. The thighs should be at right-angles to the leg, with no pressure from the seat behind the knee joint.

The ideal driving posture for a back sufferer. Ensure the buttocks are well back, the driving wheel is close to the body, and the legs are always slightly flexed. Use a good, thick, well upholstered, latex-foam cushion on seat, and at the back. Use additional cushions, if necessary.

Diag. 97. Seating postures recommended to alleviate lower lumbar pain.

8. **Avoid using the vacuum cleaner** for two weeks, as the pulling backwards and forwards of the cleaner puts some pull on the sensitive sciatic nerve, thus aggravating the condition.

9. **Diving into Swimming Pool.** This may hyperextend the spinal column, thus aggravating the condition.

10. **Straight Leg Raising.** This only stretches an already hypersensitive sciatic nerve and must be avoided.

11. **All forms of sport.** Squash, golf, tennis, hockey, football, rugby, badminton, all forms of athletics and sport which involve quick jerking movements must be discontinued until the disc has been completely detached and the nerve has settled down, usually at the end of two weeks.

12. **Driving a Car** should be avoided until the condition has cleared up. The stretching of the legs out to the pedal controls pulls on the hypersensitive spastic muscles of the lumbar spine, and the painful sciatic nerve.

13. **Avoid,** as far as possible, **coughing or sneezing.** These cause a wave of pressure of the cerebro-spinal fluid that surrounds the brain and the whole of the spinal cord. This wave will strike the hypersensitive affected nerve root and cause sharp, sudden, intense pain.

14. **Surgical corsets and plaster casts** must not be used, as this leads to a disuse atrophy in the lumbar muscles. Most patients find the use of these frustrating.

Conditions which Alleviate Sciatica

1. **Sleep on a good interior sprung mattress.** This allows the affected area to mould into the mattress, whereas the 'hard board' bed causes pressure on the tender areas. It also ensures that the spinal column is supported throughout its length.

2. **Sit on a soft seat.** Place a Dunlopillo cushion onto the chair until all symptoms have completely cleared up. This applies to a motor car seat also. Sit well into the chair with the sacrum against the back of the chair or driver's seat. Never sit on the edge of a chair with the back arching backwards. Avoid sitting on a very low chair, even if it is soft, as you will have difficulty in regaining the erect posture. Sit with the body weight onto the unaffected buttock and place a small stool under the foot of the affected side.

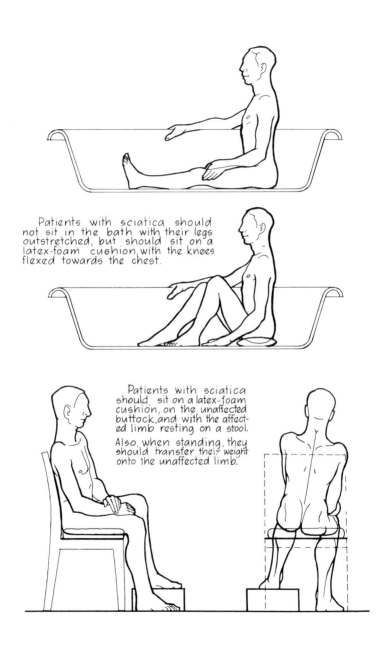

Patients with sciatica should
not sit in the bath with their legs
outstretched, but should sit on a
latex-foam cushion, with the knees
flexed towards the chest.

Patients with sciatica
should sit on a latex-foam
cushion, on the unaffected
buttock, and with the affected limb resting on a stool.

Also, when standing, they
should transfer their weight
onto the unaffected limb.

Diag. 98 Postures recommended to alleviate sciatica.

202

3. **Place a thick rubber cushion under buttocks in bath.** Never sit in the bath with the legs straight out. This will stretch the sciatic nerve and is equal to the straight leg raising test. Always bring the knees slightly upwards towards the chest.

4. **Stand with body weight onto the unaffected lower limb** and slightly flex the body laterally to this side.

5. **Walk with short steps** with the spinal column flexed laterally, slightly away from the affected side. Walking is not a good exercise and should be minimal in acute sciatic cases.

Advice to Patients Suffering from a Slipped Disc Lesion in the (Neck or) Cervical Area

What is a Slipped Disc?

A SLIPPED disc condition arises when injury, or a summation of minor injuries, causes a tear in the annular ligament that surrounds the disc. This allows the disc to prolapse through the tear and, if that disc strikes a nerve root, intense pain will ensue.

From a clinical point of view, a description of a slipped disc in the cervical region should be divided into three specific areas as the symptoms in each case are completely different. If the prolapsed disc is in the upper part of the cervical column, i.e. between C.1 and the base of the skull or between C.1/2, acute pain will be felt at the base of the skull, due to the pull on the post-occipital nerve on one side usually, or occasionally on both, leading to a post-occipital neuritis. This, in turn, may lead to a migraine-like syndrome, with pain in the region of the supra-orbital nerve or nerves in the forehead. If the prolapsed disc occurs in the mid-cervical region, the disc striking the nerve root leads to acute pain, with marked spasm of the muscles supplied by this nerve. The affected muscles in spasm will hold the neck in a fixed position pulling it towards the affected side, leading to a marked scoliosis at this level, i.e. an acute torticollis. If, however, the prolapsed disc is in the lower aspect of the cervical region i.e. between C.6/7 the disc striking a nerve root, leads to very acute pain at the base of the skull on one side or the other. It is unusual for the nerve roots on both sides to be struck at the same time. The muscles supplied by the affected nerve go into spasm which may extend partially up the neck, and may also affect muscles on the top of the shoulder and down the medial side of the shoulder blade. In most cases the brachial plexus is struck, leading to a brachial neuritis, with radiating pain. The nerves most commonly struck are the median and ulnar and this gives rise to pain extending down the arms to the fingers with possible tingling or pins and needles sensations and, at times, numbness.

Treatment

The pain and other symptoms will persist as long as the disc mechanically presses on the nerve root. This is the basic cause of the symptoms and I make it my policy to treat the cause and not the symptoms, for the latter will disappear in their own time, once the treatment has been achieved. In order to effect a permanent cure, the disc must be detached from its source of nutrient and allowed to atrophy. This I do manually under local anaesthesia, i.e 'Nerve Root Block' and, at the first treatment, non-surgical detachment of all the disc that is protruding through the tear in the annular ligament is carried out. During successive treatments, three or four in all, more disc will protrude and be detached similarly until it is all cleared away, often within one week.

During the same appointments, I gently manipulate the neck to correct the torticollis caused by muscle spasm. Audible clicks may be heard during this process but this is not the disc being 'put back', as is often thought, but the clicking of one bony facet over another. The disc is, in fact, jelly-like and cannot either be 'put back' or cause any clicking sound.

The Training Programme

Muscles that are in spasm, caused by the mechanical pressure of the disc on the nerve root supplying those muscles, are not in good tone. Thus I prescribe a training programme to regain tone in the affected muscles. The prescribed exercises must not be neglected, for the muscles must eventually be strengthened to support the head in its normal alignment. They must be performed daily with patience and perseverance especially if the condition is longstanding. It is important that the patient takes deep breaths with each movement, as oxygen is essential for muscle toning and regeneration.

206

The Training Programme for Cervical Disc Lesions

Exercise I (Cervical)

1. Stand erect with feet together.

2. Jerk the head backwards, and then forwards but only as far as the erect posture, (never bending the neck forwards).

3. Repeat 10 times.

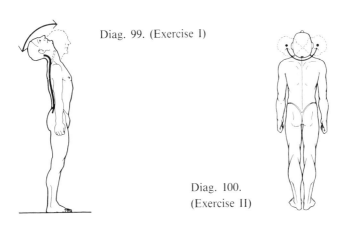

Diag. 99. (Exercise I)

Diag. 100.
(Exercise II)

Exercise II (Cervical)

1. Stand erect with feet together.

2. Hold the head backwards.

3. Rotate the head in this axis, ear to shoulder, five times to one side. Avoid bringing the head forwards beyond the shoulder point.

4. Similarly, rotate in the opposite direction five times.

5. The rotation should follow the course of the round part of a capital 'D'. The head should never be rotated round and round as this will cause dizziness.

Exercise III (Cervical)

1. Stand erect with feet together.

2. Hold the head back, looking up to the ceiling.

3. Stretch the arms out straight in front and parallel to the floor.

4. With elbow joints fixed and fists clenched rotate the stiff arms quickly backwards as in swimming breast stroke, with the shoulder blades coming together when the arms are right back.

5. Swing the stiff arms down past the body and repeat 20 times, four times a day. Take a deep breath when the arms are being raised to the horizontal plane, and exhale as the shoulder blades are brought together.

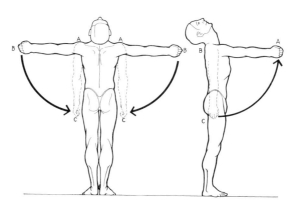

Diag. 101.

Exercise III — as well as getting the muscles of the neck in good tone, it also exercises the supra-scapular, medial scapular and the arm muscles. If there is a degree of cervical spondylosis present, exercises II and III will tone up the affected muscles and ligaments and a full range of movement will be obtained.

Exercise IV (Cervical)

1. The patient may sit or stand for this exercise.

2. With the head erect and looking forward, turn the neck slowly but firmly sideways, until the chin is in line with the top of the shoulder. Then pause for a count of five.

3. Perform the exercise five times in each direction, three or four times a day.

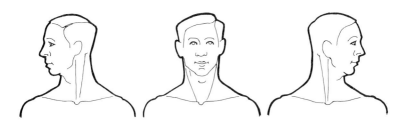

Diag. 102.

All these exercises should be carried out at least three or four times a day. Sportsmen and women, should carry out this programme every hour of the day until all symptoms have gone and the affected muscles are in first class tone. For many of my patients, I recommend that they carry out this training for a minute or two night and morning for the rest of their lives.

If the patient follows this training programme he is helping himself to get fit and he is usually cured after 10-14 days. However, in some cases (about 2-3%) symptoms can be slow to clear up, depending possibly on the length of time the patient has been suffering. Also in older age groups of patients, symptoms are somewhat slower to clear up.

It helps if the patient understands why the pain persists in some cases. When a slipped disc has been striking a nerve root for a considerable time, the nerve will have become very, very sensitive and will remain so for a time after the striking has been discontinued. In a similar way, the pain from a blow on the chin will last much longer than the actual blow and the injured area remains sensitive for some considerable time.

209

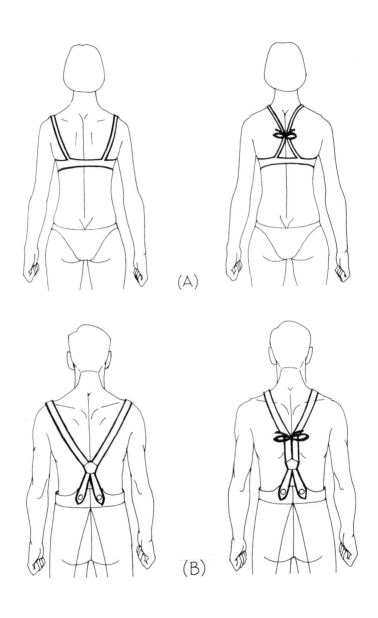

(A)

(B)

Diag. 103. Methods of alleviating brachial neuritis.

210

Conditions which Aggravate the Disc Lesions in the Neck

It is important to avoid any state that will aggravate the condition.

1. **The patient must not wear or use a surgical collar.** This leads to a disuse atrophy in the cervical muscles. The use of a cervical collar in bed only, is commonly recommended but this also should be discontinued. Not only does it cause muscle atrophy but many patients suffer from a choking feeling and often one of claustrophobia.

2. **Avoid wearing a garment which pulls the shoulder downwards.** The wearing of a garment which pulls the shoulder downwards will, in particular, aggravate the brachial neuritis by pulling on the hypersensitive nerve roots. Female patients must ensure that they wear a correctly fitting bra. The straps of this should be pulled medially towards the base of the neck, either by tying the straps at the back together or by cutting the straps at the back and re-stitching them two inches nearer the midline. If male patients wear braces they should avoid pull on the points of the shoulders by fixing the anterior clips towards the midline or by tying the straps at the back together.

3. **Avoid,** as far as possible, **coughing or sneezing.** These cause a wave pressure of the cerebro-spinal fluid that surrounds the brain and the whole of the spinal cord. This wave will strike the hypersensitive affected nerve root and cause sharp, sudden, intense pain.

Conditions which Alleviate Brachial Neuritis

1. An important factor in helping to relieve the symptoms of brachial neuritis is to choose and arrange the **pillows in bed** during sleep. Pillows must be used to keep the cervical column in a straight line with the remainder of the spinal column. The pillows should be placed to fill in the square between the side of the head and the shoulder when the patient lies on his side. Care should be taken that the pillows are high enough to prevent the head falling towards the pillow, but not too high, so that the head is overflexed leading to acute strain and pain. Usually two pillows give the satisfactory height. The same principle applies if the patient prefers to lie on his back. A small 9″ x 4″ bolster may be used to support the neck in this position. I recommend the use of down-filled pillows for all patients suffering from pain in the neck.

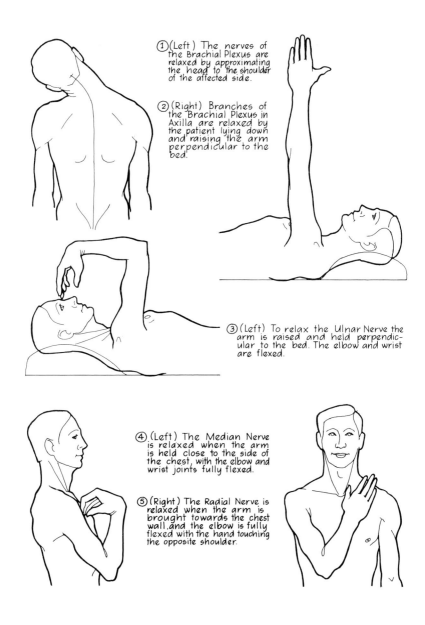

① (Left) The nerves of the Brachial Plexus are relaxed by approximating the head to the shoulder of the affected side.

② (Right) Branches of the Brachial Plexus in Axilla are relaxed by the patient lying down and raising the arm perpendicular to the bed.

③ (Left) To relax the Ulnar Nerve the arm is raised and held perpendicular to the bed. The elbow and wrist are flexed.

④ (Left) The Median Nerve is relaxed when the arm is held close to the side of the chest, with the elbow and wrist joints fully flexed.

⑤ (Right) The Radial Nerve is relaxed when the arm is brought towards the chest wall, and the elbow is fully flexed with the hand touching the opposite shoulder.

Diag. 104. Methods of relaxing the nerves of the brachial plexus.

212

2. **Hold the shoulder upwards** on the affected side by using a temporary sling. Alternatively, the hand may be placed in a buttoned jacket in a Napoleon-like fashion. This will alleviate pull on the affected hypersensitive nerve roots.

Advice to Patients Suffering from a Slipped Disc Lesion in the Dorsal or Thoracic Region

What is a Slipped Disc?

A SLIPPED disc condition arises when injury, or a summation of minor injuries, causes a tear in the annular ligament which surrounds the disc. This allows the disc to prolapse through this tear and if that disc strikes a nerve root, intense pain will ensue. If the slipped disc is in the thoracic or dorsal region, the dorsal nerve struck will give rise to pain radiating round the chest to the anterior wall. When this occurs on the left side of the chest, particularly at the level of D.7/8, the symptoms are quite similar to those of a heart attack. Once a disc has struck a nerve root, pain will continue in the hypersensitive nerve, leading to a spasm of all muscles supplied by that nerve. The muscles in spasm, will pull the spinal column towards them, giving rise to a moderate scoliosis, or lateral twisting of the spinal column to the affected side. The muscles in spasm may also increase the normal dorsal kyphosis, giving rise to a hump-like deformity or rounding of the back.

Treatment

The cause of the pain and other symptoms is the mechanical pressure of the disc on a nerve root and I make it my policy to treat this basic cause first and then the symptoms will gradually disappear once the treatment has been achieved. To effect a permanent cure the disc must be detached from its source of nutrient and allowed to atrophy. I detach the disc manually, following my non-surgical technique of the detachment of the disc, under local anaesthesia. At the first treatment, I detach only that portion of the disc that is protruding through the tear in the annular ligament. On successive treatments, usually three or four, more disc will protrude during the gentle activity of the patient and I detach it similarly. It should be pointed out that the detachment of the disc in the thoracic area is the most difficult to carry out, because of the interference of the rib articulation with the spinal column, which prevents straightforward access to the disc for detachment.

During the same appointments, I commence to correct, by manipulation, the deformity caused by muscle spasm. Audible clicks may be heard during this process but this is not the disc being 'put back' as is generally supposed, but the clicking of one bony facet over another. The disc is, in fact, jelly-like and cannot be 'put back' or cause any clicking sound.

The Training Programme

Muscles that are in spasm, caused by the mechanical pressure of the disc on the nerve root supplying those muscles, are not in good tone. Thus I prescribe a training programme to regain tone in the affected muscles. The prescribed exercises must not be neglected but be performed daily with patience and perseverance, especially if the condition is longstanding. The muscles must be strengthened to support the spinal column in its normal alignment. It must be remembered that muscles will quickly lose their tone if they are not kept active and that oxygen is essential for muscle building, so deep breaths must be taken, when performing the exercises.

Training Programme for Dorsal Disc Lesions

Exercise I (Dorsal)

1. Stand in the erect posture, with feet together.

2. With stiff elbow and wrist joints and clenched fists stretch the arms out sideways at shoulder level, parallel to the floor.

3. Rotate the chest as far as it will go, from side to side. This, in turn, rotates the dorsal or thoracic vertebrae.

4. Repeat 20 times in each direction, four times a day.

5. Breathe in and out with each movement.

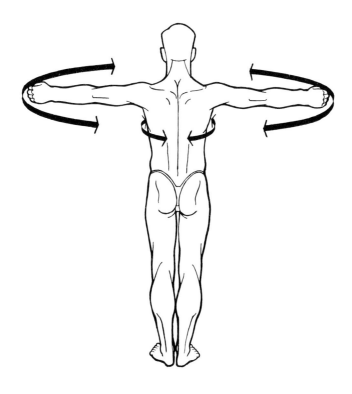

Diag. 105.

Exercise II (Dorsal)

1. Stand in the erect posture with feet together.

2. With stiff elbows and wrist joints and clenched fists stretch the arms out sideways at shoulder level, parallel to the floor.

3. Lower one arm, bending at the waist with the other pointing upwards, still with the arm straight and in line with the tip of the shoulders.

4. Holding this posture, whip the arms first one way and then the other.

5. Repeat 20 times in each direction.

6. Repeat 20 further times with the chest flexed at the waist in the opposite direction.

7. Inhale and exhale regularly to prevent overtiring of the muscles.

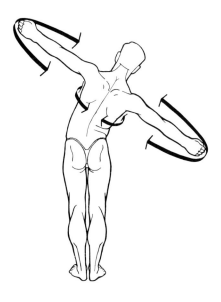

Diag. 106.

Exercise III (Dorsal)

1. The patient may either sit or stand.

2. Clasp hands on the top of the head, with elbows raised as high as possible.

3. Swing the chest from side to side for about 2″, extending upwards with every movement.

4. Repeat 20 times in each direction.

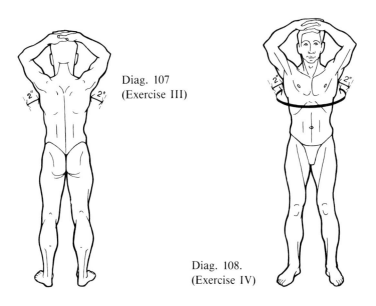

Diag. 107
(Exercise III)

Diag. 108.
(Exercise IV)

Exercise IV (Dorsal)

1. Adopt the same posture as for Exercise III.

2. Rotate the chest, bending 2″ in all directions.

3. Repeat 20 times one way, and 20 times the other.

219

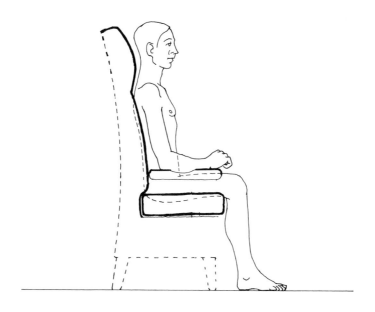

① The chair should be relatively upright with a well sprung back, to support the contour of the whole spinal column. It should also have a relatively high seat.

② To obtain relief from lower back pain, patients should sit with their buttocks into the back of the seat and their feet on the floor. They should also ensure that the thighs are at right angles to the leg and that the seat cushion causes no pressure behind the knee joints.

③ Most seat cushions of easy chairs and couches are too deep for the length of the adult thigh, and often the seats are too low. These two factors, especially in combination, mean that the individual has great difficulty in regaining the erect posture.

Diag. 109. Recommended posture requirements for easy chairs.

EXERCISES II and IV involve a rotating movement and were devised to allow compression of the column, thus encouraging further portions of disc to protrude through the tear in the annular ligament, the sharp edges of which will automatically cut off the protruding disc. Exercise III has the effect of muscle toning traction, causing extension of the spinal column in the dorsal area.

If the patient follows this training programme he is helping me to help himself get fit and he is usually cured after 10-14 days. However, in some cases (about 2-3%), symptoms can be slow to clear depending, possibly, on the length of time the patient has been suffering. Also in older age groups, patients' symptoms are somewhat slower to clear up.

It helps if the patient understands why the pain persists in some cases. When a slipped disc has been striking a nerve root for a considerable time the nerve will have become very, very sensitive and will remain so for a time after the striking has been discontinued. In a similar way, the pain from a blow on the chin will last much longer than the actual blow and the injured area remains sensitive for some considerable time.

It is important to avoid any state that will aggravate the condition and the following advice is given as a guideline to the patient to help him to cope with these persisting symptoms, explaining which activities will cause distress and those that will alleviate discomfort.

Activities which Aggravate a Slipped Dorsal Disc

1. **Quick jerky movements** must be avoided, and this includes all forms of sport, which should be discontinued for 2-3 weeks.

2. **Avoid heavy lifts.**

3. **Avoid toe touching.**

4. **Avoid diving,** but swimming is a useful exercise.

5. **Avoid,** as far as possible, **coughing or sneezing.** These cause a wave pressure of the cerebro-spinal fluid that surrounds the brain and the whole of the spinal cord. This wave will strike the hypersensitive affected nerve root and cause sharp, sudden, intense pain.

6. **Avoid the hardboard bed** and do not sleep on the affected side.

Activities which Alleviate a Slipped Dorsal Disc

1. **Shallow breathing** will prevent expansion of the chest wall and thus will minimise the movement of the rib at the site of the disc lesion.

2. **Sit on a straight backed chair** with the chest expanded and the shoulders well back to prevent pressure on the affected area. The back of the chair should be soft. Lean backwards on to unaffected side.

3. Carry out the full training programme four times a day. Chronic cases should perform these exercises every two hours.

THE AUTHOR

MR. ALEXANDER WALKER-NADDELL was born in Glasgow and studied medicine at Glasgow University, qualifying just before the outbreak of the Second World War. After serving with great distinction and gallantry with the Commandos during the war, and later with Strategic Command he resumed his studies and became a Fellow of the Royal Faculty of Physicians and Surgeons (qua Surgeon) and later a Fellow of the Royal College of Surgeons.

He worked first as a General Surgeon, later specialising in orthopaedic and neuro-surgery, at the Glasgow Royal Infirmary and Killearn Hospital and it was during this period that the major part of his research into the anatomy of the spinal column took place.

About 30 years ago, he set up in private practice in the West End of Glasgow and achieved so much success with his unique treatment of the slipped disc, that his reputation in this sphere has spread not only throughout the United Kingdom but overseas as well. Many patients come from the United States, Canada, the Middle East and even as far as from Australia. Sportsmen and women, in particular, continuously seek his help and many have publicly expressed their gratitude for being able to continue in their sporting careers due to his treatment.

Quite apart from his success in his professional life he has received many other honours reflecting his varied activities. He was made a Knight of Justice of the Most Venerable Order of St. John of Jerusalem in recognition of his work for that Order. For services to his City he was appointed Deputy Lieutenant of Glasgow and for over twenty years he was first a J.P. and later acted as a District Court Judge. Since the war, as Colonel of his Regiment, he has been actively associated with the Army as well as taking part in Defence Re-organisation and military training and strategy. In recognition of this he was awarded the Emergency Reserve Decoration.

Throughout his life he has been passionately interested in all kinds of sport, especially golf, rugby and boxing. In his youth he was a keen athlete, especially noted for his sprinting, and he represented his University many times in his student days. It was perhaps his active participation in sport that first led so many sportsmen and women to come to him for help. A diagnosis of a slipped disc to them meant that, either the continuous intense pain or the variable results of surgery to cure it, would inevitably have adverse consequences on their game and ruin their sporting careers. A good sportsman or woman, often at the peak of achievement, would be lost for ever. After treatment by the special technique for the non-surgical detachment of the slipped disc, these players have been able to continue to play their sport often within a fortnight and many top players, golfers, footballers, rugby players, etc., at this very moment owe their present positions to the treatment of Mr. Walker-Naddell. The ability to cure this group of patients, combining, as it does, his medical skills with his involvement in the world of sport has perhaps provided some of the most rewarding experiences of his professional life.